The Wonder of What We Eat
Workbook

Activities and Reflections to Help Kids Build Healthy Habits and a Positive Relationship with Food

Written By:
Ritu Saluja-Sharma MD
Dylan Sharma

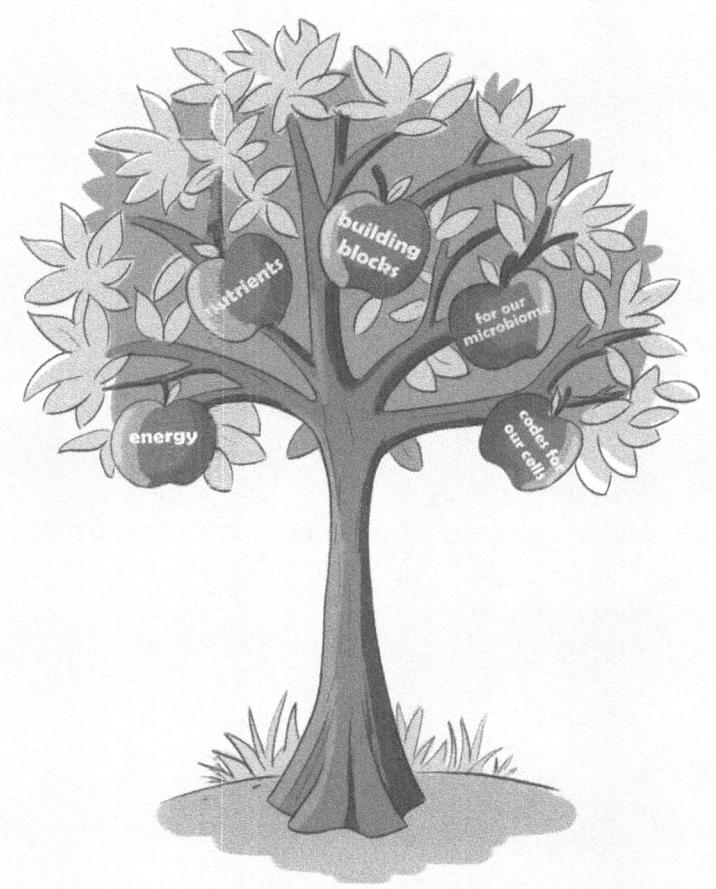

The Wonder of What We Eat Workbook
By Ritu Saluja-Sharma MD and Dylan Sharma

Cover Illustration by Navdeep Kaur Komal

A companion workbook to:
**The Wonder of What We Eat:
How Our Incredible Food, Our Incredible Bodies, And Our Incredible Planet Are Connected**
By Ritu Saluja-Sharma MD

Published by Head Heart Hands LLC
Headhearthandsmd.com

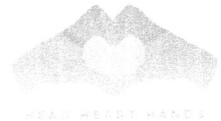

Copyright © 2025 Ritu Saluja-Sharma and Dylan Sharma

All rights reserved.
No part of this publication may be reproduced, distributed, or transmitted in any form or by any means, including photocopying, recording or other electronic or mechanical methods, without the prior written permission of the publisher. For permissions, contact: headhearthandsmd@gmail.com.

Disclaimer
The content of this book is for general informational purposes only. Each person's physical, emotional, and spiritual condition is unique. The instruction in this book is not meant to be used, nor should it be used, to diagnose or treat any medical condition or to replace the services of your physician or other healthcare provider. The advice and strategies contained in the book may not be suitable for all readers. Neither the author, publisher, nor any of their employees or representatives guarantees the accuracy of information in this book or its usefulness to a particular reader, nor are they responsible for any damage or negative consequence that may result from any treatment, action taken, or inaction by any person reading or following the information in this book.

ISBN: 979-8-9990505-2-6

CONTENTS

Introduction — i

LESSON 1:	Health Is Not Just Numbers on a Scale	01
LESSON 2:	Our Bodies Are Incredible	04
LESSON 3:	Food Is Not Just Calories	07
LESSON 4:	Matching Macronutrients for the Win	10
LESSON 5:	Sorting Carbohydrates	13
LESSON 6:	Brain Friendly Fats	17
LESSON 7:	Matching Miraculous Micronutrients	20
LESSON 8:	The Remarkable Rainbow of Phytonutrients	25
LESSON 9:	Your Miraculous Microbiome	30
LESSON 10:	Sending Signals to Your Cells	33
LESSON 11:	Getting Familiar with Food Labels	36
LESSON 12:	Searching for Sugar on Labels!	40
LESSON 13:	Spotting Artificial Sweeteners	44
LESSON 14:	Fiber for the Win	48
LESSON 15:	Investigating Ingredient Lists	52
LESSON 16:	Finding Fat on Labels	56
LESSON 17:	Sleuthing Sodium on Labels	59
LESSON 18:	Uncovering Ultra-Processed Foods	62
LESSON 19:	Foods Pretending to Be Healthy with a Health Halo	66
LESSON 20:	Creating an Incredible Plate	69
LESSON 21:	The Power of Protein From Plants	73
LESSON 22:	Nourish Your Body and Heal the Earth	76
LESSON 23:	The Media and Our Health	80
LESSON 24:	My Weekly Wins!	83
LESSON 25:	Share What You Learned!	89
LESSON 26:	Making Decisions	92
LESSON 27:	Setting a SMART Goal	95
LESSON 28:	Recognizing Valid & Reliable Resources	98
LESSON 29:	Helping Yourself, Helping Others, and Helping the Earth	103
LESSON 30:	Next Stop – the Grocery Shop!	106
	Answer Key	111

INTRODUCTION

Welcome to **The Wonder of What We Eat Workbook**!
You're about to learn some pretty amazing things—about your food, your body, and how powerful your everyday choices can be.

This isn't about rules, feeling bad about what you eat, or being "perfect."
It's about discovering how your amazing food can fuel your brain, boost your mood, and help your body do incredible things—like grow stronger, think clearly, sleep better, and feel your best.

In this workbook, you'll get to:

Use what you have learned to solve real-life challenges

Think about your own habits and goals

Build confidence and skills that will last a lifetime

This workbook goes along with the book ***The Wonder of What We Eat: How Our Incredible Food, Our Incredible Bodies, and Our Incredible Planet Are Connected***.

If you've read it already—great! If you haven't read it yet, don't worry—you'll still learn so much right here! In order for you to get the most out of this workbook, you can read the book while doing this workbook and refer to it during the lessons!

Think of this as your space to explore, reflect, and take action.
And remember: You don't need to be an expert or do everything perfectly.
Just be curious, honest, and open to learning new things.

You're the expert on YOU.
This workbook will help you feel strong, smart, and confident as you take care of your health in a way that works for YOU.

Let's get started!

LESSON 1:
HEALTH IS NOT JUST NUMBERS ON A SCALE

> Most adults have unfortunately been taught that **their weight (the number on the scale) is the way to see if they are healthy.** But that's not true! Just like food is more than the number of calories, **our health is more than the number on our scale**. Our body's health depends on our habits—what we eat, how we sleep, how much we move, and how we care for ourselves.

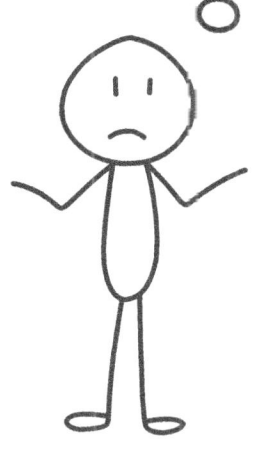

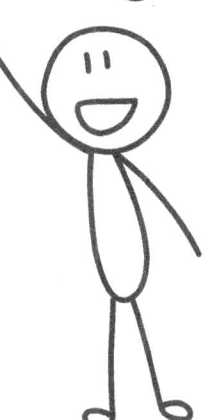

A   B

WORKSHEET 1
HEALTH IS NOT JUST NUMBERS ON A SCALE

1. Character A is focused only on weight. What might they think about all day? How might they feel about their body? What might they eat or avoid?

   ----

2. Character B focuses on habits. How might they think about their body? What might they eat? What might they do to feel strong and healthy?

   ----

3. Who is more likely to feel better about their body and their choices?

WORKSHEET 1
HEALTH IS NOT JUST NUMBERS ON A SCALE

4. Why might people think that they should focus on weight? Where do you think they learned this?

_____
_____
_____
_____

5. Why is focusing on health habits and nourishment better than just focusing on weight?

_____
_____
_____

6. What does real health feel like to you?

_____
_____
_____
_____

LESSON 2:
OUR BODIES ARE INCREDIBLE

> **Our body contains 30 trillion cells.** Every day, we replace over 330 billion of them! Our heart beats 100,000 times a day. Our immune system protects us. Our brain sends signals through nerve cells. **Our bodies are doing amazing things every second!**

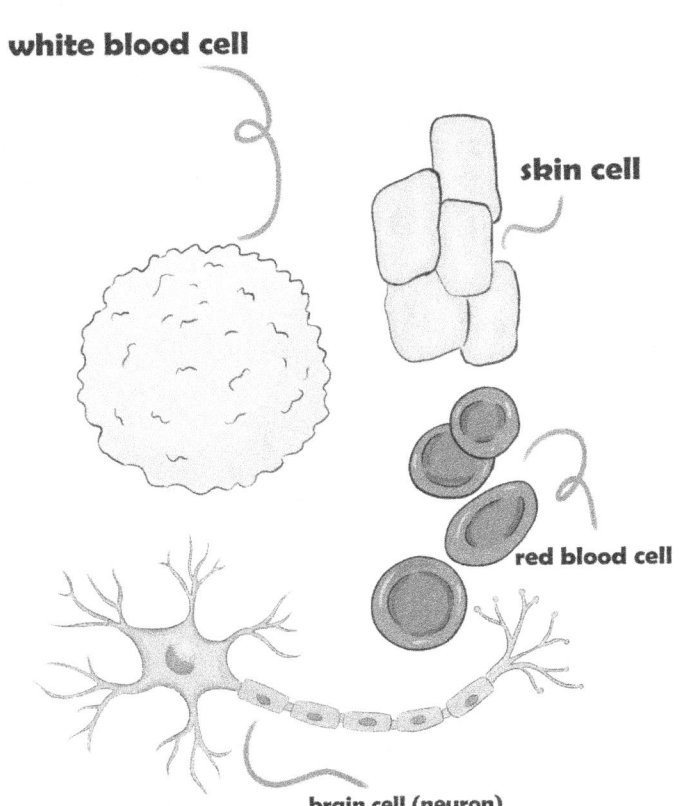

WORKSHEET 2
OUR BODIES ARE INCREDIBLE

Match each body part with its amazing function in your body:

1. HEART

2. BRAIN

3. MUSCLES

4. LUNGS

5. STOMACH & INTESTINES

6. CELLS

7. NERVES

A. Sends lightning-fast messages to help you move, think, feel, and remember.

B. Pumps blood and oxygen to your entire body—beats over 100,000 times a day!

C. Breathe in oxygen and get rid of carbon dioxide—about 20,000 breaths a day!

D. Power every move you make—from jumping to chewing—over 600 in your body!

E. Tiny building blocks—trillions of them! They help you grow, heal, and stay strong.

F. Carry messages at over 250 mph from your brain to your body (and back)!

G. Break down food, absorb nutrients, and give you the energy to run, think, and play.

WORKSHEET 2
OUR BODIES ARE INCREDIBLE

1. What's something incredible your body can do?

---

2. What foods do you eat that help your body stay strong?

---

3. "My body is amazing because..."

LESSON 3:

FOOD IS NOT JUST CALORIES

> Calories are just one measure of energy. **But food is so much more than energy!** Food is building blocks, micronutrients, food for our microbiome, and messages/instructions for our body.
>
> A food with fewer calories isn't always the healthier choice.

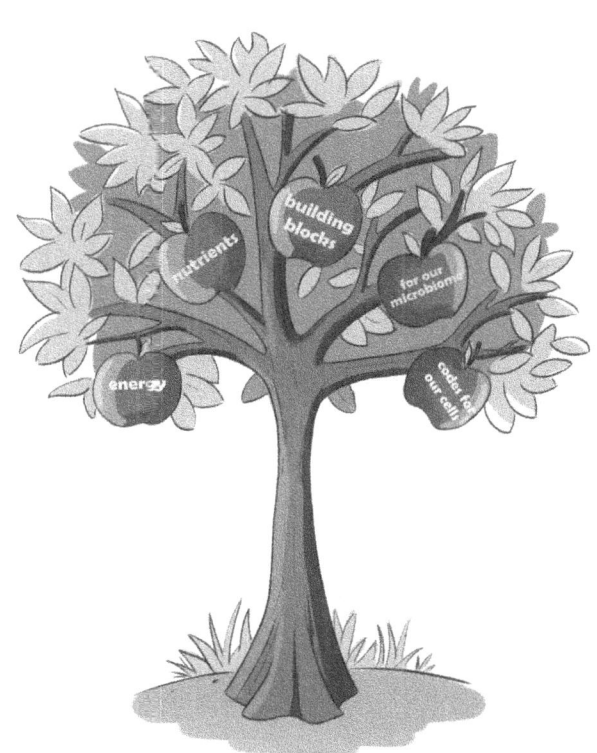

Food is energy.
Food is nutrients that allow our cells to function.
Food is the building blocks of our body.
Food is food for our microbiome.
Food is messages/codes for our cells.

WORKSHEET 3

FOOD IS NOT JUST CALORIES

COMPARE TWO SNACKS

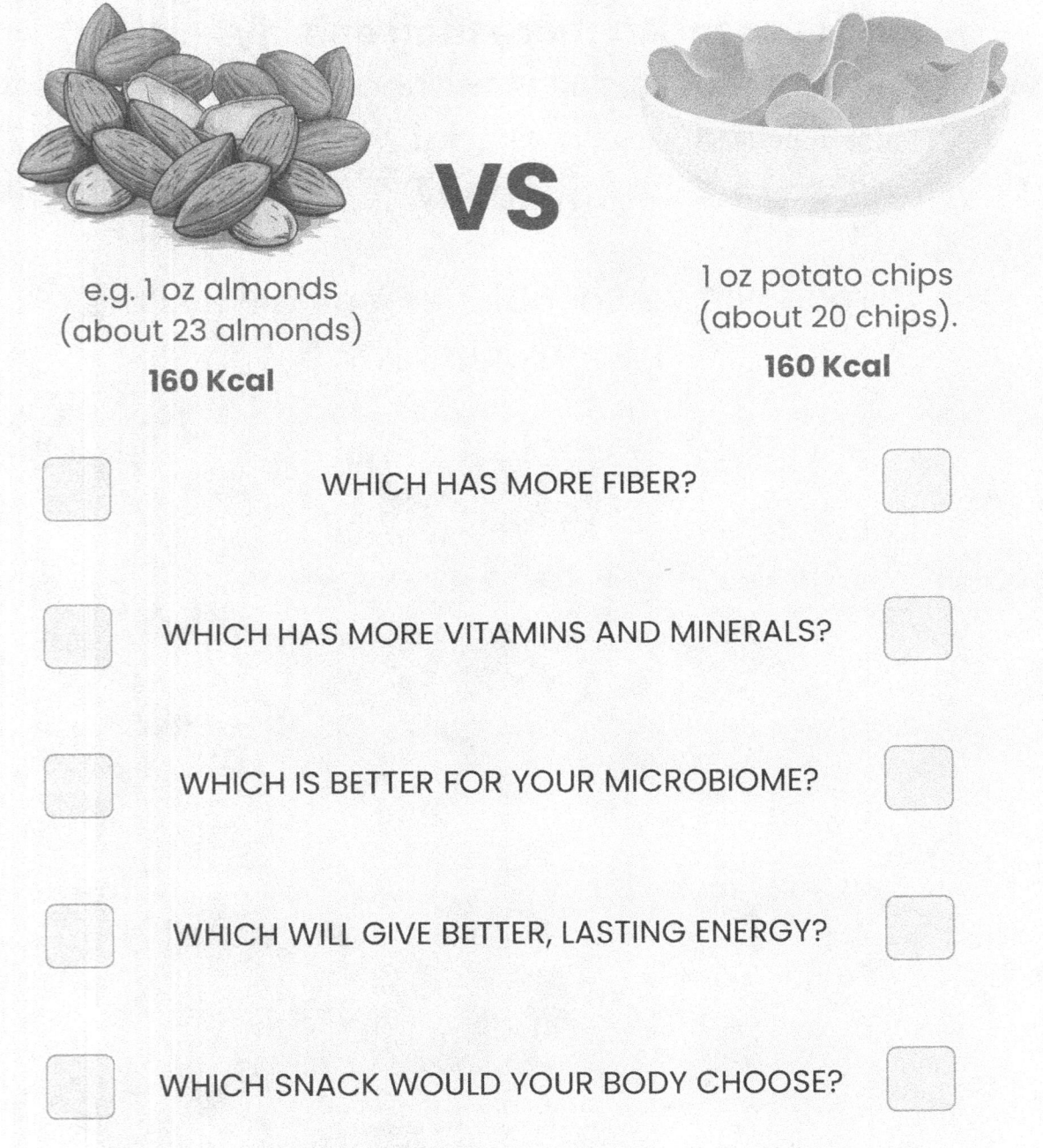

e.g. 1 oz almonds
(about 23 almonds)
160 Kcal

1 oz potato chips
(about 20 chips).
160 Kcal

☐ WHICH HAS MORE FIBER? ☐

☐ WHICH HAS MORE VITAMINS AND MINERALS? ☐

☐ WHICH IS BETTER FOR YOUR MICROBIOME? ☐

☐ WHICH WILL GIVE BETTER, LASTING ENERGY? ☐

☐ WHICH SNACK WOULD YOUR BODY CHOOSE? ☐

WORKSHEET 3
FOOD IS NOT JUST CALORIES

1. Why might people think low-calorie means healthy?

_____
_____
_____
_____

2. Which snack (the almonds or the chips) would you want before soccer practice or a test?

_____
_____
_____
_____

3. "Food is more than a number of calories because..."

_____
_____
_____
_____

LESSON 4:
MATCHING MACRONUTRIENTS FOR THE WIN

> Our bodies need macronutrients—carbohydrates, proteins, and fats—to survive and thrive.
>
> Carbohydrates are our body's preferred source of energy. Carbohydrates include foods like fruits, vegetables, beans, lentils, rice, bread, pasta, and oats.
>
> Protein builds muscle and repairs cells. Protein can be found in meat, dairy, and eggs, but also in plants, including beans, lentils, peas, edamame, tofu, nuts, and seeds.
>
> Fats help our brain, cells, and hormones. Fat can be found in lots of food, including oil, butter, meat, dairy, nuts, nut butters, seeds, and avocados.

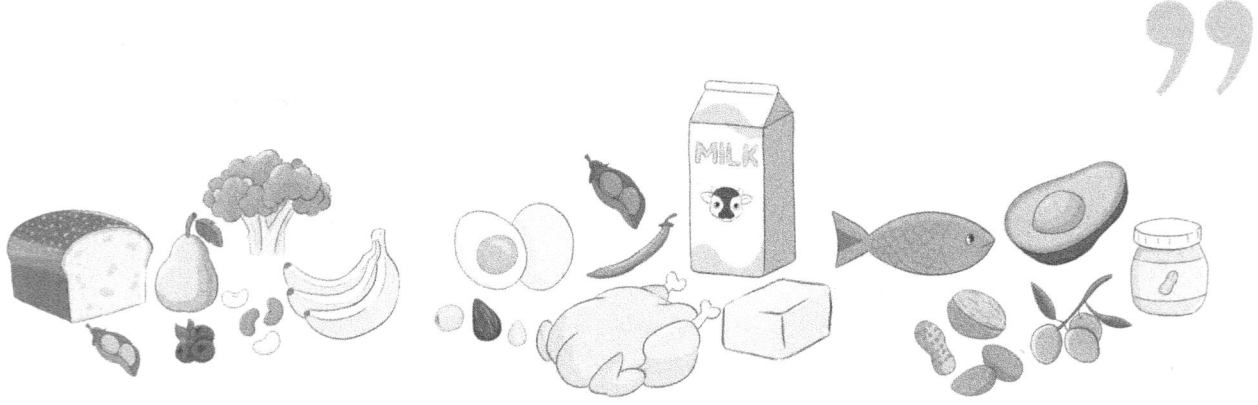

Carbohydrates   Proteins   Fats

WORKSHEET 4
MATCHING MACRONUTRIENTS FOR THE WIN

Sort the foods into the correct columns:
(Hint: Some foods can be in more than one column).

Foods:	Carbohydrates	Protein	Healthy Fat
Oatmeal			
Bananas			
Nuts			
Yogurt			
Tofu			
Salmon			
Chicken			
Avocados			
Beans			
Whole grain bread			
Apples			
Peanut butter			
Seeds			
Olive oil			

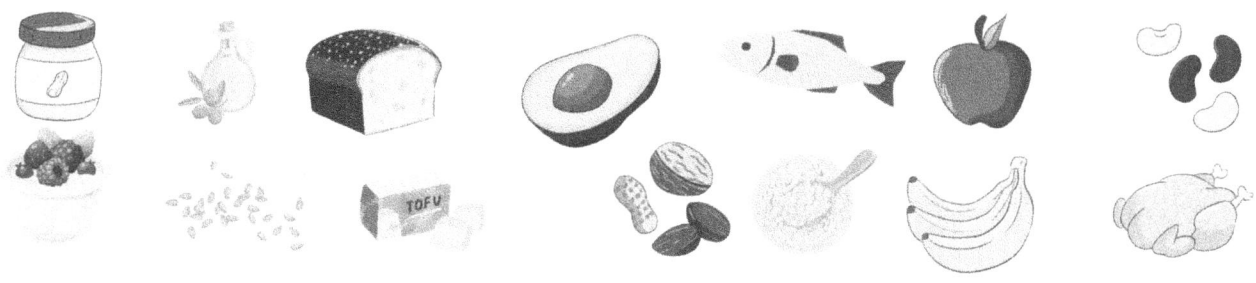

WORKSHEET 4
MATCHING MACRONUTRIENTS FOR THE WIN

1. What would happen if you didn't eat enough protein?

   _____
   _____
   _____
   _____

2. Which nutrients do you think your body uses most when you're playing sports?

   _____
   _____
   _____
   _____

3. "A healthy food I like that has protein is…"

   _____
   _____
   _____
   _____

LESSON 5:
SORTING CARBOHYDRATES (SIMPLE VS. COMPLEX CARBOHYDRATES)

"

Simple carbohydrates (like candy, white bread, white rice, sweet drinks, and most packaged snacks) can be quickly digested because most of the fiber and nutrients are removed when the food is created in factories. Eating simple carbohydrates can give us a burst of energy, but then can cause an energy crash.

On the other hand, complex carbohydrates (like fruits, vegetables, beans, lentils, and whole grains like rolled oats and quinoa) take longer to digest because of the natural fiber in them. This is why complex carbohydrates give us stable, long-lasting energy. Eating mostly complex carbohydrates instead of simple carbohydrates can even have a positive effect on our mood, our concentration, and our memory.

Complex carbohydrates are the carbohydrates nature designed for us to eat!

"

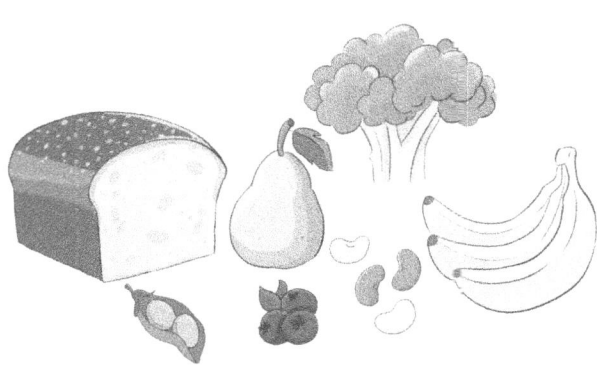

Complex Carbohydrates

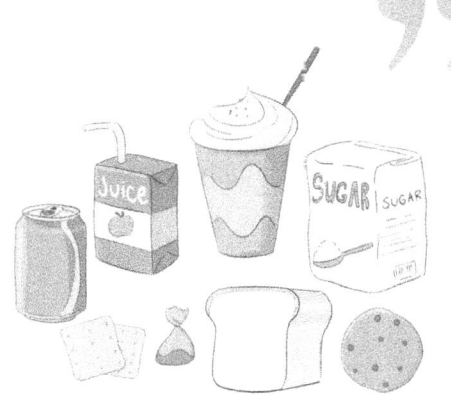

Simple Carbohydrates

WORKSHEET 5
SORTING CARBOHYDRATES (SIMPLE VS. COMPLEX CARBOHYDRATES)

Identify which foods are complex carbohydrates and which foods are simple carbohydrates. Place a ✓ for all of the complex carbohydrates, and an X for all of the simple carbohydrates.

✓ Complex Carbohydrates   ✗ Simple Carbohydrates

Food		Food	
Rolled oats	☐	Soda	☐
Cookies	☐	Broccoli	☐
Apples	☐	White bread	☐
Fruit Juice	☐	White Pasta	☐
Lentils	☐	White Rice	☐
Quinoa	☐	Whole grain bread	☐
Doughnuts	☐	Whole Wheat Pasta	☐
Sugary Cereal	☐	Steel Cut Oats	☐
		Oranges	☐

WORKSHEET 5
SORTING CARBOHYDRATES (SIMPLE VS. COMPLEX CARBOHYDRATES)

1. Why might it feel better to have stable, long lasting energy, rather than energy spikes and crashes?

_____
_____
_____
_____
_____
_____
_____

2. How do you think energy spikes and crashes might affect your mood and ability to concentrate?

_____
_____
_____
_____
_____
_____
_____

WORKSHEET 5
SORTING CARBOHYDRATES (SIMPLE VS. COMPLEX CARBOHYDRATES)

3. How can you tell which foods will give lasting energy?

   _____
   _____
   _____
   _____
   _____
   _____
   _____

4. "Some foods that helps me stay energized and focused are..."

   _____
   _____
   _____
   _____
   _____
   _____
   _____

LESSON 6:

BRAIN FRIENDLY FATS

"Fat is important for your body and brain! But not all types of fat are the same.

The healthy fats in nuts, seeds, avocados, olives, and fish help your brain think clearly and your cells stay strong.

Other fats like trans fats or too much saturated fat, can hurt your heart, your blood vessels and your energy. Trans fats can be found in packaged foods (like microwave popcorn, refrigerated doughs, pre-made baked goods), and fried foods.

Saturated fat is solid at room temperature, like the fat in butter. You also find saturated fat in fatty pieces of meat (especially red meat), cheese, whole milk, and in packaged baked goods that use saturated plant fats such as palm oil and coconut oil"

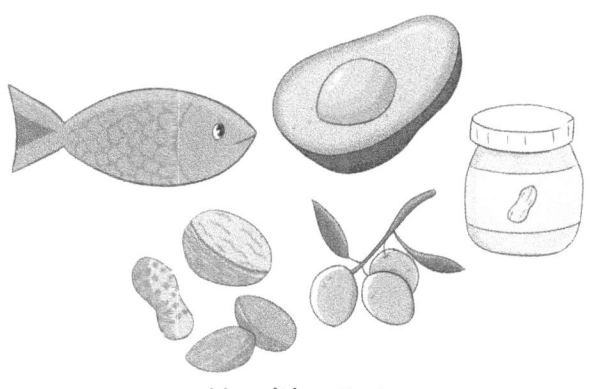

Healthy Fats

WORKSHEET 6

BRAIN FRIENDLY FATS

"Sort the fat!" game: Place an X in the boxes for the fats your BRAIN would choose.

- Avocados ☐
- Olive oil ☐
- Walnuts ☐
- Salmon ☐
- Fried Chips ☐
- Packaged Pastries ☐
- Cheeseburgers ☐
- Pumpkin seeds ☐
- French fries ☐

WORKSHEET 6

BRAIN FRIENDLY FATS

1. Did you know your brain is made of mostly fat? How does that make you feel about fat? Does this make you want to choose healthier fats and eat less saturated fats and trans fats?

_____
_____
_____
_____

2. What are some ways you can get more brain-healthy fats?

_____
_____
_____
_____

3. "One healthy fat I can eat more of is..."

_____
_____
_____
_____

LESSON 7:
MATCHING MIRACULOUS MICRONUTRIENTS

"Micronutrients (vitamins and minerals) help your body perform over 1 billion billion (1 quintillion) chemical reactions every second! These nutrients keep your bones, skin, brain, and immune system strong—and they come mostly from whole foods like fruits, veggies, beans, seeds. lean meats, and whole grains."

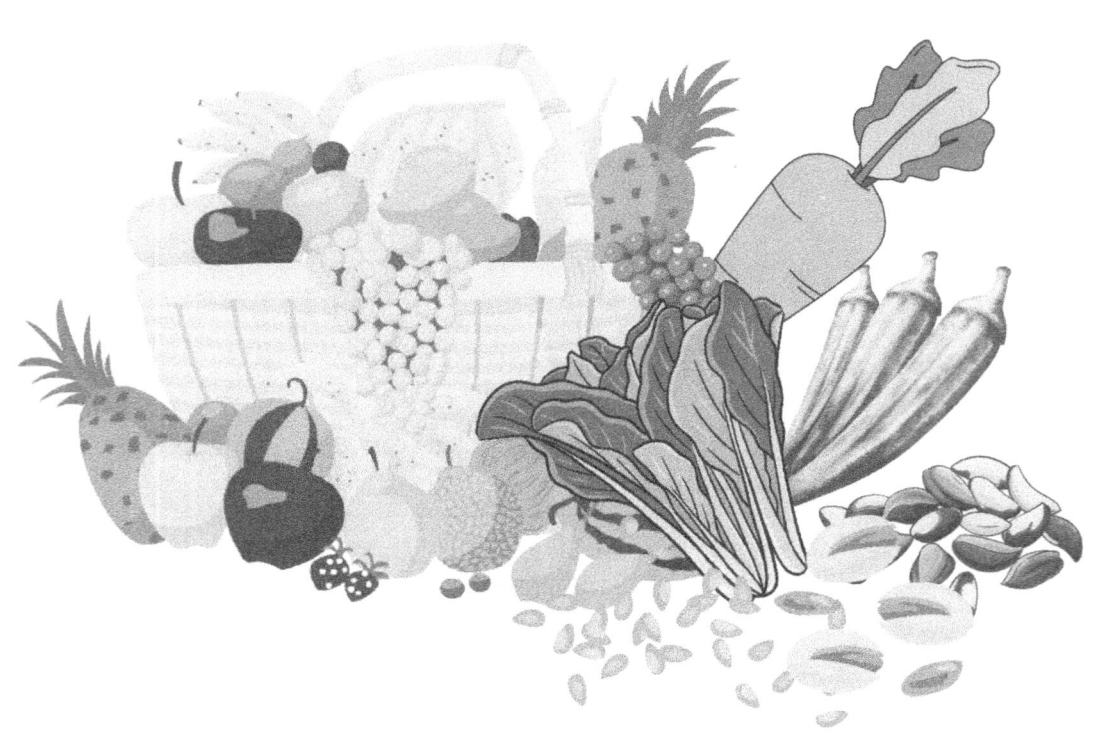

LESSON 7
MIRACULOUS MICRONUTRIENT CHART

Nutrient	Function	Sources
Calcium	Builds strong bones and teeth and keeps your muscles moving.	Broccoli | Almonds | Tofu | Milk | Fortified soy milk
Iron	Helps your body make blood, which carries oxygen around your body to give you energy.	Spinach | Lentils | Meat | Fish | Tofu | Pumpkin Seeds
Magnesium	Helps muscles work, keeps bones strong, and supports energy production.	Green Leafy Vegetables | Pumpkin Seeds | Black Beans | Almonds
Potassium	Helps your muscles move and keeps your heart beating steadily.	Bananas | Sweet potatoes | Beans | Avocados
Vitamin A	Keeps your eyes sharp, helps you grow, and protects you from getting sick.	Carrots | Sweet potatoes | Spinach | Kale | Cantaloupe
Vitamin B1 (Thiamine)	Turns food into energy so you can run, jump, and play, and keeps your nerves healthy.	Whole grains | Beans | Nuts | Seeds
Vitamin B12 (Cobalamin)	Keeps your nerves and blood healthy and helps make your DNA.	Fish | Dairy Foods | Eggs
Vitamin B2 (Riboflavin)	Helps you get energy from food and keeps your skin and eyes strong.	Milk | Yogurt | Spinach | Mushrooms
Vitamin B3 (Niacin)	Helps your body break down food and use it for energy.	Peanuts | Mushrooms | Whole grains | Peas

LESSON 7
MIRACULOUS MICRONUTRIENT CHART

Nutrient	Function	Sources
Vitamin B5 (Pantothenic Acid)	Supports making energy and important hormones your body needs.	Avocados | Sweet potatoes | Broccoli | Whole grains
Vitamin B6 (Pyridoxine)	Helps your brain think clearly and makes important blood cells.	Bananas | Chickpeas | Spinach | Potatoes
Vitamin B7 (Biotin)	Helps your body use energy and keeps your skin, hair, and nails healthy.	Almonds | Sweet potatoes | Spinach | Eggs
Vitamin B9 (Folate)	Builds new cells to help you grow and heal faster.	Spinach | Broccoli | Lentils | Oranges
Vitamin C	Strengthens your immune system and helps your body heal cuts and bruises.	Oranges | Strawberries | Bell peppers | Broccoli
Vitamin D	Helps you absorb calcium to build strong bones and teeth. Helps your immune system and brain stay strong and healthy.	Sunlight | Mushrooms | Fish | Fortified Soy Milk | Fortified Dairy Products
Vitamin E	Protects your cells and keeps your skin and eyes healthy.	Almonds | Sunflower seeds | Spinach | Avocados
Vitamin K	Helps your blood clot if you get a cut and keeps your bones strong.	Broccoli | Spinach | Kale | Green beans
Zinc	Strengthens your immune system and helps heal wounds quickly.	Pumpkin Seeds | Cashews | Chickpeas | Lentils

WORKSHEET 7
MATCHING MIRACULOUS MICRONUTRIENTS

Match each micronutrient to the food source it's found in, and then to its function in the body:

Micronutrient	Food Source	Function
Vitamin C	Oranges	Immune system and healing wounds
Magnesium	sun/fish	Muscles, bones, and energy
Iron	Broccoli, spinach, kale, green beans	Healthy blood
Vitamin D	leafy greens, nuts, seeds	Helps your blood clot
Vitamin K	spinach, lentils, meat	Immune system, brain & bones

23

WORKSHEET 7
MATCHING MIRACULOUS MICRONUTRIENTS

1. What are some new foods you can add to your plate, in order to eat more micronutrients?

_____

_____

_____

2. Why is having a strong immune system important?

_____

_____

_____

3. "Some new foods I can eat that will give my body vitamins are..."

_____

_____

_____

LESSON 8:
THE REMARKABLE RAINBOW OF PHYTONUTRIENTS

"Phytonutrients are powerful plant chemicals that protect your body and brain. Carotenoids (yellow, orange, and red veggies) help your eyes. Anthocyanins (purple and blue foods) help your brain. Eating all the colors of the rainbow helps your body stay healthy!"

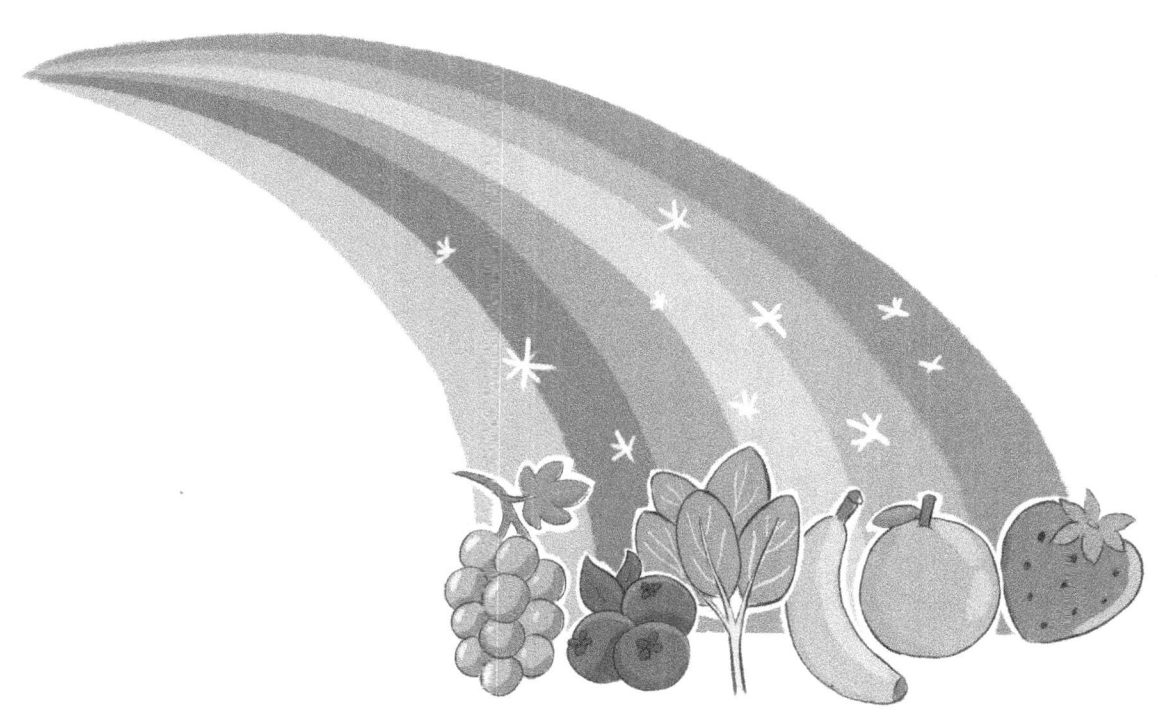

WORKSHEET 8
PHYTONUTRIENT CHART

RED
Lycopene:
Protects your heart and helps keep your skin healthy

 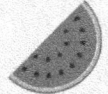

ORANGE
Beta-Carotene
Keeps your eye sharp and immune system strong

 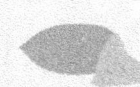

YELLOW
Lutein & Zeaxanthin
Protect your eyes and help your brain stay sharp

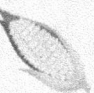 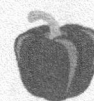 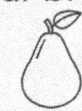

GREEN
Sulforaphane:
Protects your cells and helps your body get rid of harmful toxins

 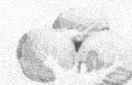 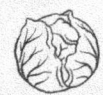

BLUE & PURPLE
Anthocyanins:
Help your memory and protect your brain

WHITE
Allicin
Boosts your immune system and helps fight germs

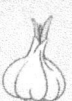 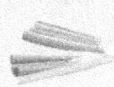

WORKSHEET 8
THE REMARKABLE RAINBOW OF PHYTONUTRIENTS

Color in a rainbow food chart with 6 colors. Use the phytonutrient rainbow chart to list a few foods that you like from each color

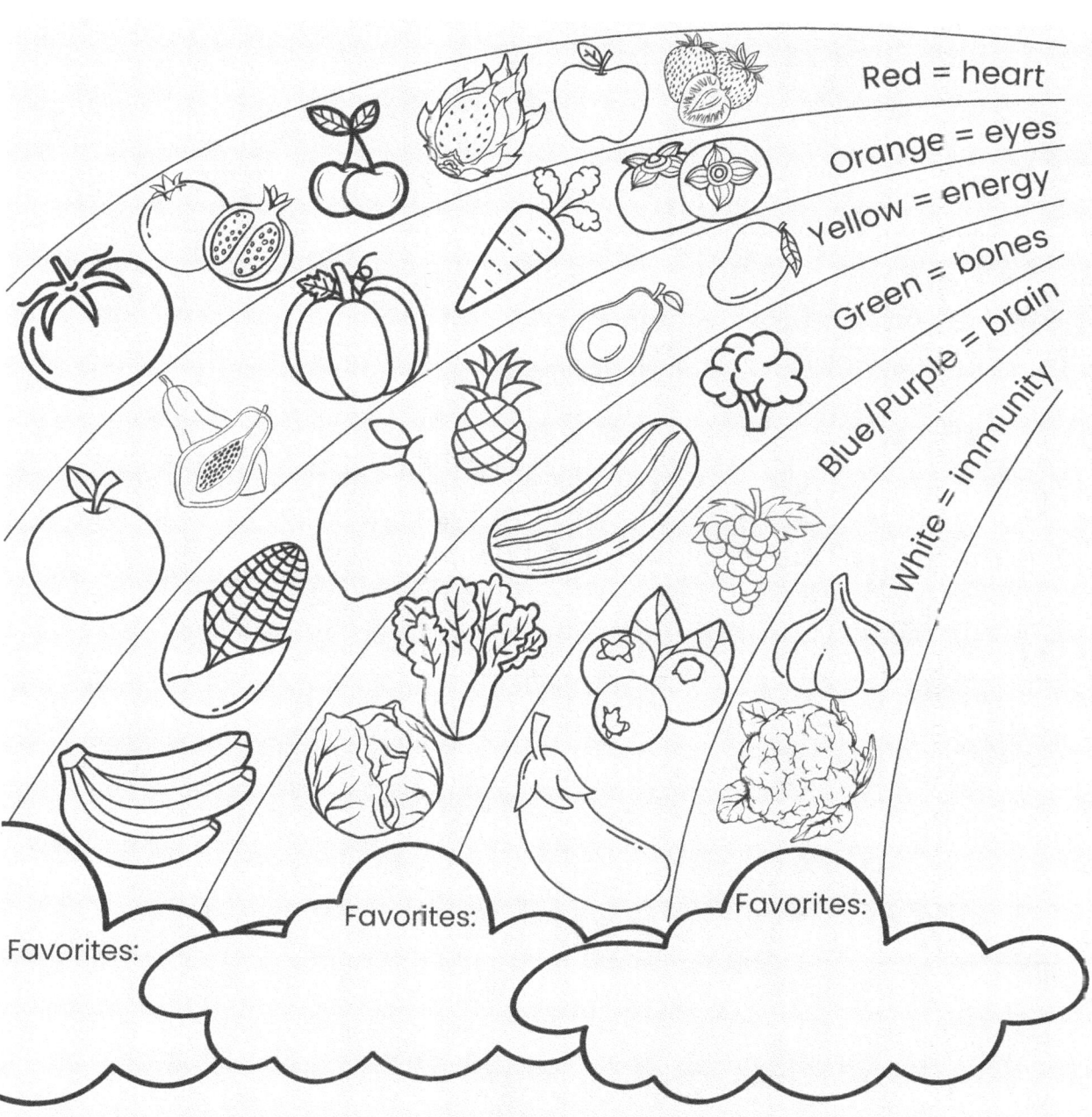

WORKSHEET 8
THE REMARKABLE RAINBOW OF PHYTONUTRIENTS

1. What color foods did you eat today?

_____
_____
_____
_____
_____
_____
_____

2. Is there a rainbow color you don't eat very often?

_____
_____
_____
_____
_____
_____
_____

WORKSHEET 8
THE REMARKABLE RAINBOW OF PHYTONUTRIENTS

3. "Tomorrow I want to try a new _____ color food!" Here are some foods I can add to eat more colors...

----

4. What are some foods you can add to try to "eat the rainbow" for every day this week!

Sunday:

Monday:

Tuesday:

Wednesday:

Thursday:

Friday:

Saturday:

LESSON 9:

YOUR MIRACULOUS MICROBIOME

"You're not eating alone—your gut microbiome is eating with you! These trillions of microbes help your immune system, digestion, and even your mood. Your microbiome loves fiber-rich foods like fruits, veggies, beans, oats, and nuts. Your microbiome does not like food with lots of sugar or chemicals."

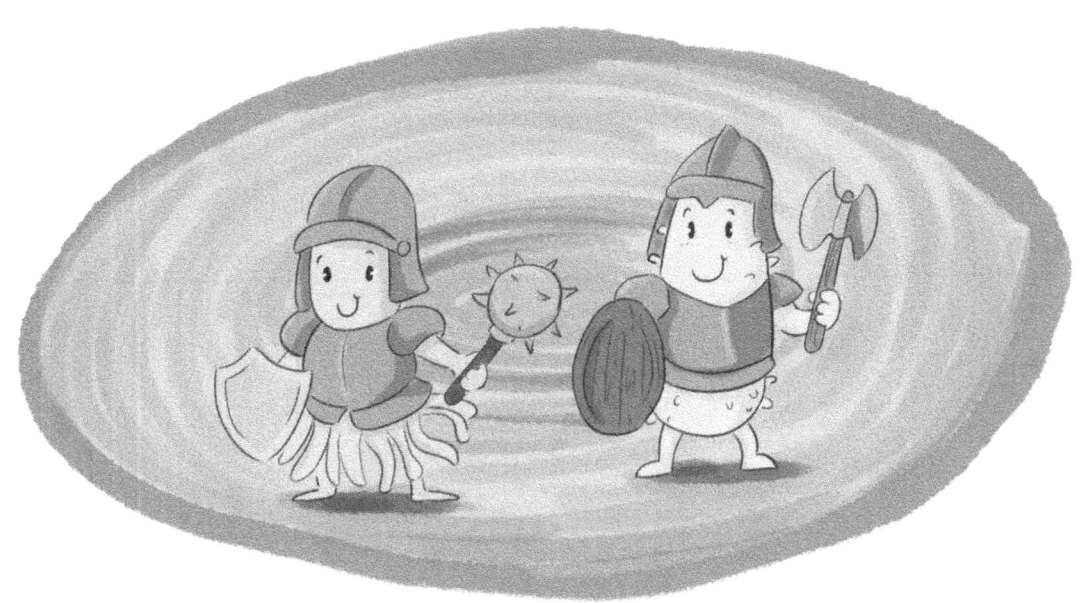

WORKSHEET 9

YOUR MIRACULOUS MICROBIOME

Place a ✓ for which foods you microbiome would wcnt you to eat.

- ☐ Blueberries
- ☐ Yogurt
- ☐ Rolled Oats
- ☐ Beans
- ☐ Onions
- ☐ Sugar free gatorade
- ☐ Doughnuts
- ☐ Gummy bears
- ☐ Garlic
- ☐ Asparagus
- ☐ Diet Soda
- ☐ Apples
- ☐ Lentils
- ☐ Potato Chips
- ☐ Quinoa
- ☐ White Bread

WORKSHEET 9

YOUR MIRACULOUS MICROBIOME

1. What are some foods that you can add to your plate that have fiber?

_____
_____
_____
_____

2. Why is it important that you feed your microbiome the fiber rich food it loves?

_____
_____
_____
_____

3. "Today I fed my microbiome by eating..."

_____
_____
_____
_____

LESSON 10:

SENDING SIGNALS TO YOUR CELLS

> Your DNA is like an instruction manual. Food acts like a highlighter that turns certain genes on or off. When you eat healthy food, you can send good messages to your body—like grow strong, heal better, or stay focused.

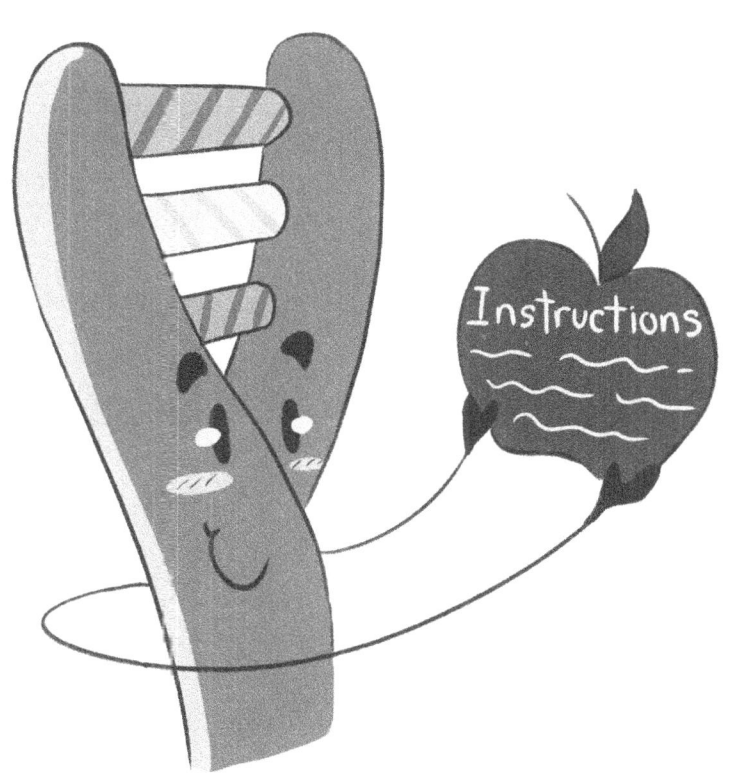

WORKSHEET 10

SENDING SIGNALS TO YOUR CELLS

Match each food to the message it sends to your body:

Food	Message
Diet soda	Whole fruit filled with phytonutrients sends good messages to your genes.
Beans	Simple carbohydrates digested quickly because there is no fiber. Stomach sends messages to your brain that you need more food.
Pretzels	Artificial sweeteners send messages to your brain to crave more sugar.
Raspberries and blueberries	Digested slowly because of the fiber. Stomach sends messages to your brain that you feel satisfied and full.
Apple juice	All of the fiber taken out of the fruit, and mostly just sugar left. Quick blood sugar spike sends a message to your pancreas to release a lot of insulin.
Broccoli	Cruciferous vegetable with lots of phytonutrients and fiber. Microbiome is happy and sends happy messages to your brain.

WORKSHEET 10

SENDING SIGNALS TO YOUR CELLS

1. What kind of messages do you want your food to send to your body?

_____
_____
_____
_____
_____
_____
_____

2. Now that you know that your food sends messages, how does this change the way you think about eating?

_____
_____
_____
_____
_____
_____
_____

LESSON 11:

GETTING FAMILIAR WITH FOOD LABELS

> Sadly, most adults never learned to read food labels properly. They often only look at calories, but calories don't tell us if food gives lasting energy, helps our microbiome, or sends healthy messages to our cells. A better approach is to look at the fiber, sugar, protein, sodium, and ingredients.

WORKSHEET 11

GETTING FAMILIAR WITH FOOD LABELS

Compare the sugar, fiber, protein, sodium and ingredients for these 2 kinds of bread. Which has more of each? (Hint: Make sure to also look at the serving size, so you can accurately compare the two kinds of bread.)

White Bread:

Nutrition Facts

10 servings per container

Serving size	2 slice

Amount per serving

Calories 140

	% Daily Value*
Total Fat 1.5g	2%
Saturated Fat 0.0g	0%
Trans Fat 0.0g	
Cholesterol 0.0mg	0%
Sodium 180.0mg	8%
Total Carbohydrates 29.0g	11%
Dietary Fiber 3.0g	11%
Total Sugars 5.0g	
Protein 5.0g	10%

* The % Daily Value (DV) tells you how much a nutrient in a serving of food contributes to a daily diet. 2,000 calories a day is used for general nutrition advice.

INGREDIENTS: Unbleached Enriched Flour (Wheat Flour, Malted Barley Flour, Niacin, Reduced Iron, Thiamin Mononitrate, Riboflavin, Folic Acid), Water, Sugar, Yeast, Contains 2% or Less of Each of the Following: Calcium Carbonate, Wheat Gluten, Soybean Oil, Salt, Dough Conditioners (Contains One or More of the Following: Sodium Stearoyl Lactylate, Calcium Stearoyl Lactylate, Monoglycerides, Mono-and Diglycerides, Distilled Monoglycerides, Calcium Peroxide, Calcium Iodate, DATEM, Ethoxylated Mono-and Diglycerides, Enzymes, Ascorbic Acid), Vinegar, Monocalcium Phosphate, Citric Acid, Cholecalciferol (Vitamin D3), Soy Lecithin, Calcium Propionate (to Retard Spoilage).

Sugar:
Fiber:
Protein:
Sodium:
Ingredients:

Whole Grain Ezekiel Bread:

Nutrition Facts

20 servings per container

Serving size	1 slice

Amount per serving

Calories 80

	% Daily Value*
Total Fat 0.5g	1%
Saturated Fat 0.0g	0%
Trans Fat 0.0g	
Cholesterol 0.0mg	0%
Sodium 75.0mg	3%
Total Carbohydrates 15.0g	5%
Dietary Fiber 3.0g	11%
Total Sugars 0.0g	
Protein 5.0g	10%

* The % Daily Value (DV) tells you how much a nutrient in a serving of food contributes to a daily diet. 2,000 calories a day is used for general nutrition advice.

INGREDIENTS: Organic Sprouted Wheat, Filtered Water, Organic Sprouted Barley, Organic Sprouted Millet, Organic Malted Barley, Organic Sprouted Lentils, Organic Sprouted Soybeans, Organic Sprouted Spelt, Yeast, Organic Wheat Gluten, Sea Salt.

Sugar:
Fiber:
Protein:
Sodium:
Ingredients:

WORKSHEET 11

GETTING FAMILIAR WITH FOOD LABELS

Were you surprised by the differences in these 2 types of bread?

Which one has more sugar per slice?

Which one has more protein per slice?

Which one has more fiber per slice?

Which one has less sodium per slice?

How are the ingredients different between the 2 types of bread?

Circle which bread is a healthier choice. Explain why.

Why is it important to look at the serving size when comparing labels?

WORKSHEET 11

GETTING FAMILIAR WITH FOOD LABELS

1. What surprised you when you looked at the ingredient lists?

   ----

2. What's more helpful than calories when choosing food?

   ----

3. Next time I look at a label, I'll check for...

LESSON 12:

SEARCHING FOR SUGAR ON LABELS!

Too much sugar is unhealthy for your microbiome and can cause your blood sugar to go way up and then crash. This can send unhealthy messages to your cells.
By looking closely at food labels, you can find out how much sugar is in your food.

It is important to look at the total amount of sugar, the amount of added sugar, and for sugar in the ingredient list. Ideally, it is best to choose foods that are low in sugar, especially added sugar.

Eating a piece of whole fruit, which contains natural sugars but no added sugar, is a great option to satisfy your sweet tooth.
It is recommended that kids and teens eat less than 25 grams of added sugar per day. Most kids eat way more than that, because a lot of food companies sneak added sugar into almost everything. Even foods that don't taste super sweet can have hidden added sugars. On labels, added sugar can be listed with lots of different names like corn syrup, dextrose, and cane juice.

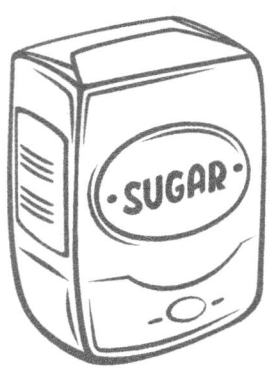 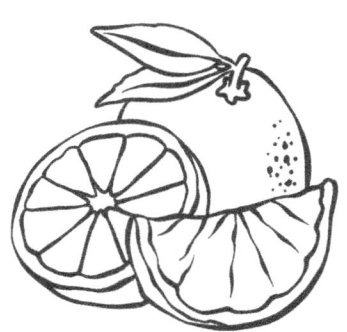

WORKSHEET 12

SEARCHING FOR SUGAR ON LABELS!

Find the hidden names of sugar:

```
A Y U I O P H K F J X H H J J Z F D N G E
C G G I D J H J G A M V J H B R Q B N X V
F G A N F F G H F F G G S F U G D G C G A
X D S V D S S F X D F B J C X A S A E G P
M B N D E X T R O S E G T N E A Y A S F O
Q A N L N N X F S R A O B A F E F F C F R
W D L B Z B E Z X Z S R Q S N Q D R R G A
E D D T H J X C C E R G J O S Q S F C D T
F F D Z O V B Z T S F R H T R E D X U S E
S S E X T S J Z D A R D T E S A F S S G D
F G S A D D E J V C R F K S F S F D A F C
M O L A S S E S H U Q W Y G T A D E S B A
Q W E R T Y F Z S H S E S Z X C D W S Z N
F R U I T J U I C E C O N C E N T R A T E
A S D F G H J K L Q W T Y U J D Q V A H J
C O R N S Y R U P S F R D T G F D F F J U
F V E T Y S S H F D J F G Q S F S F F G I
G D D G G F D G D J H F G H B H T H F F C
L D K F K U Y D T D T D T Y D R G F H F E
H I G H F R U C T O S E C O R N S Y R U P
```

Agave Nectar

Corn syrup

Dextrose

Evaporated cane juice

Fruit juice concentrate

High fructose corn syrup

Honey

Maltose

Molasses

Sucrose

WORKSHEET 12

SEARCHING FOR SUGAR ON LABELS!

1. Why might food companies add sugar to so many foods?

　

2. How can too much sugar make you feel tired or cranky?

WORKSHEET 12

SEARCHING FOR SUGAR ON LABELS!

3. How can you tell if the food you're eating has hidden sugar?

----

4. Next time I feel like eating something sweet, here are some fruits that I can choose...

LESSON 13:
SPOTTING ARTIFICIAL SWEETENERS

"Artificial sweeteners are fake sugars, that were often invented in a chemistry lab. Food companies try to make people believe that artificial sweeteners are healthy choices—but unfortunately, they can be harmful to our bodies also. Artificial sweeteners can send unhealthy messages to our cells, and they can hurt our microbiome. They can also even send messages to our brain to make us crave sugar. Rather than choosing foods and drinks with artificial sweeteners, it is best to choose naturally sweet foods like fruit and to drink water instead."

WORKSHEET 13

SPOTTING ARTIFICIAL SWEETENERS

Find the hidden artificial sweeteners:

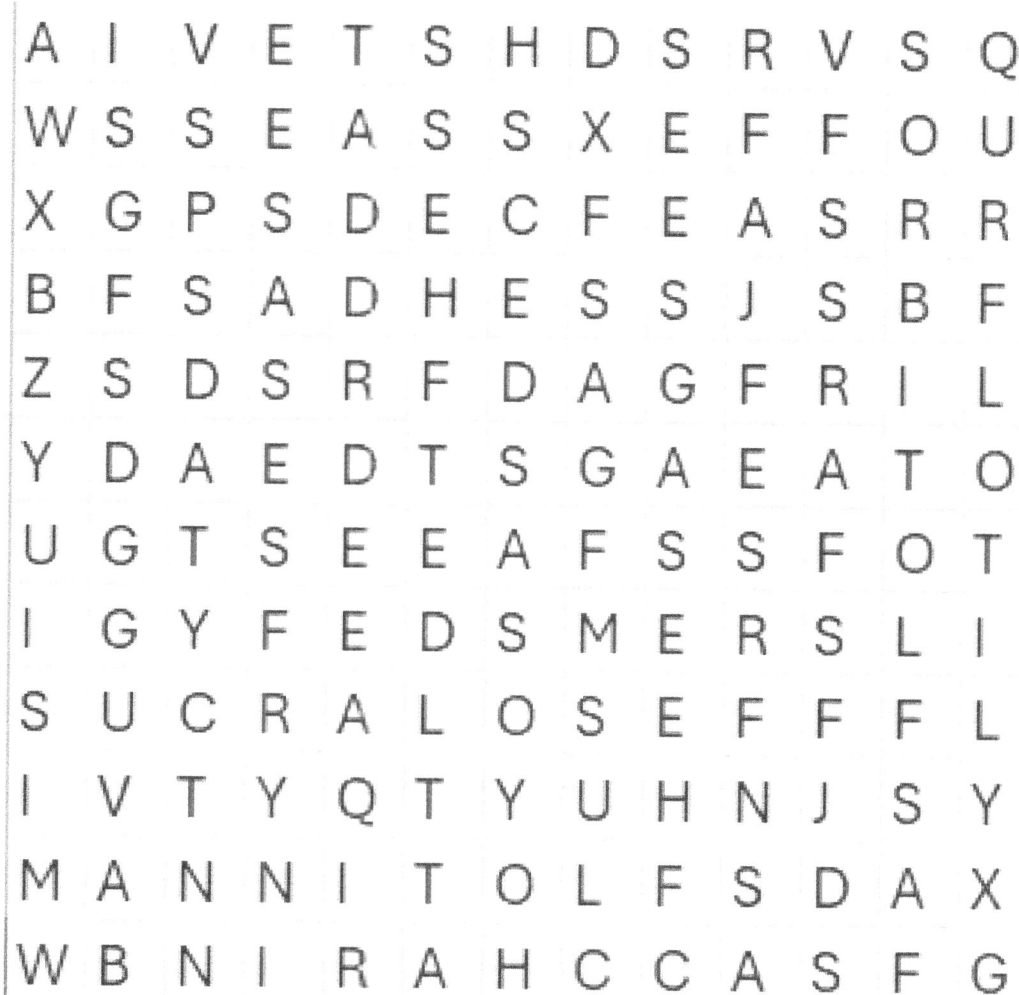

Words to find (Pronunciation in parenthesis):

Aspartame (AS-par-tame)
Sorbitol (SOR-bih-tol)
Mannitol (MAN-ih-tol)
Stevia (STEE-vee-uh)
Xylitol (ZY-lih-tol)
Sucralose (SOO-kruh-lohs)
Saccharin (SAK-uh-rin)

WORKSHEET 13

SPOTTING ARTIFICIAL SWEETENERS

1. Why might food companies create "diet" and "sugar free" products, and use artificial sweeteners?

2. Why is it misleading when foods are labeled as "healthy" or "diet" foods, but they contain artificial sweeteners?

WORKSHEET 13

SPOTTING ARTIFICIAL SWEETENERS

3. How can artificial sweeteners affect your body?

_____
_____
_____
_____
_____
_____
_____

4. What can you look for on the label to see if the food you are eating has hidden artificial sweeteners?

_____
_____
_____
_____
_____
_____
_____

LESSON 14:

FIBER FOR THE WIN

> "Fiber is only found in plants and is your microbiome's favorite food. Most ultra-processed foods are stripped of fiber. When you eat fiber at every meal, it helps your microbes thrive. Fiber also helps your digestion. When you eat enough fiber, you are better able to get rid of waste (poop)."

How Much Fiber Do Kids Need?

One way to estimate how much fiber you need is to take your age and add 5 or 10 to it. For example:

- A 5-year-old should aim to get at least 10–15 grams (g) of fiber every day.
- A 10-year old should aim to get at least 15–20 grams (g) of fiber a day.
- A 15-year-old should aim to get at least 20–25 grams (g) of fiber a day.
- Adults should aim to get at least 25-30 grams of fiber a day

These amounts are the minimum amount of fiber that is recommended! It is best to aim for much more!

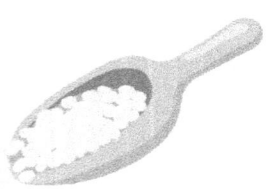 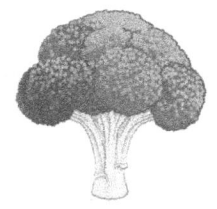 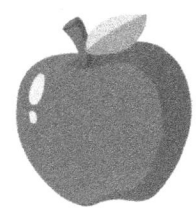 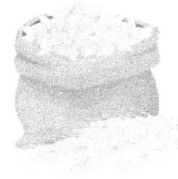

LESSON 14:

FIBER FOR THE WIN

FIBER IN VEGETABLES:

Peas (1 cup)	9 grams
Lima Beans (1 cup)	13 grams
Broccoli (1 cup)	5 grams
Edamame (1 cup)	8 grams
Brussel Sprouts (1 cup)	4 grams
Sweet potato (1 cup)	5 grams
Cauliflower (1 cup)	2.1 grams
Okra (1 cup)	3.2 grams

FIBER IN FRUIT:

Raspberries (1 cup)	9 grams
Blueberries (1 cup)	13 grams
Pear (1 medium)	5 grams
Apple with skin (1 medium)	8 grams
Avocado (1 cup)	8 grams
Banana (1 cup sliced)	3.9 grams
Strawberries (1 cup)	3.3 grams
Mango (1 medium)	5 grams

FIBER IN NUTS AND SEEDS:

Almonds (1 oz):	9 grams
Pistachios (1oz):	13 grams
Walnuts (1 oz):	5 grams
Pecans (1 oz):	8 grams
Sunflower Seeds (1/4 cup):	3 grams
Flaxseeds (1 tablespoon):	2.8 grams
Chia Seeds (1 oz):	10 grams

FIBER IN LEGUMES:

Black beans (1 cup):	15 grams
Chick peas boiled (1 cup):	12 grams
Kidney Beans cooked (1 cup):	14 grams
Pinto Beans cooked (1 cup):	15 grams
Navy Beans cooked (1 cup):	19 grams
Lentils boiled (1 cup):	16 grams
Lentil Pasta (3 oz):	9 grams

Create a list of what you ate today. Using the chart above to estimate your fiber intake, do you think that you ate enough fiber?

FOOD	FIBER	FOOD	FIBER
1._____	____grams	5._____	____grams
2._____	____grams	6._____	____grams
3._____	____grams	7._____	____grams
4._____	____grams	8._____	____grams

WORKSHEET 14:

FIBER FOR THE WIN

Using the fiber chart, list some foods that you can add to your meals that contain fiber. Create a sample meal plan for breakfast, lunch, and dinner for one day so that you eat enough fiber.

Fiber Rich Foods I Want to Eat....

Breakfast

Lunch

Dinner

WORKSHEET 14:

FIBER FOR THE WIN

1. Why is it important to eat fiber?

   _____
   _____
   _____
   _____

2. What happens when we don't eat enough fiber?

   _____
   _____
   _____
   _____

3. What are some fiber-rich foods that you can add to your breakfast, lunch, snack, and dinner.

   _____
   _____
   _____
   _____

LESSON 15:

INVESTIGATING INGREDIENT LISTS

> Ultra-processed foods often have long lists of ingredients that sound like they were made in a lab, not a kitchen. A good rule: If there are a lot of words you don't recognize or can't pronounce, it's probably an ultra-processed food.

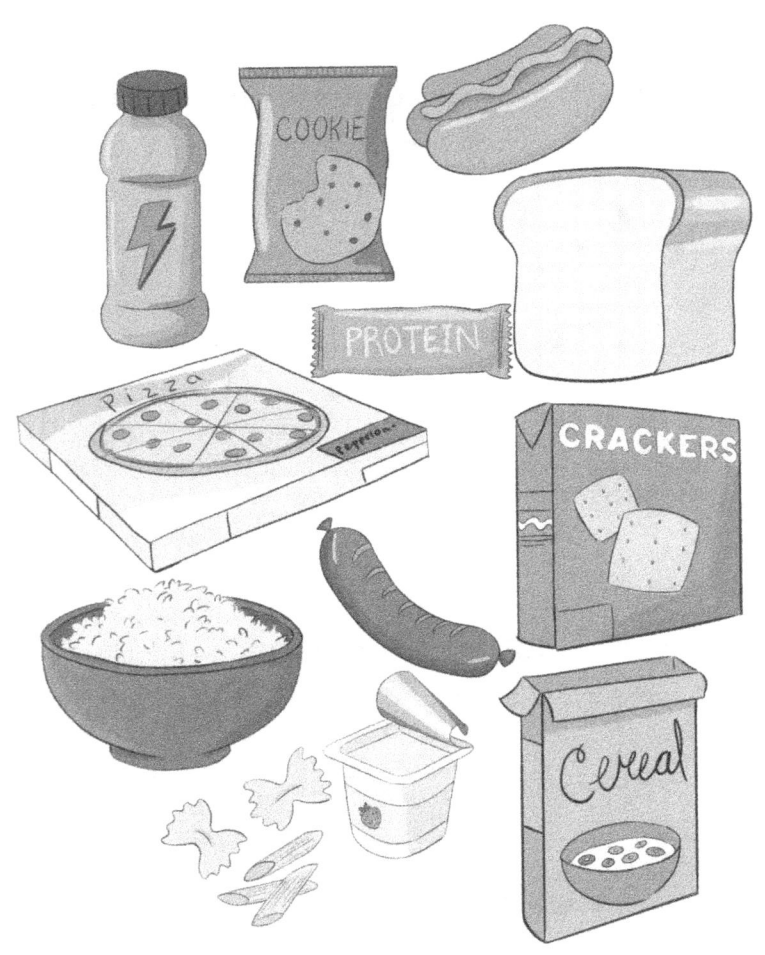

WORKSHEET 15:

INVESTIGATING INGREDIENT LISTS

Look closely at the ingredient lists for each of these foods.

✓ Place a check for the foods with ingredients you might find in a normal kitchen.

✗ Place an X for the foods with ingredients you don't recognize.

Vanilla Berry Yogurt Cup

Nutrition Facts

4 servings per container
Serving size: 1

Amount per serving
Calories 140

	% Daily Value*
Total Fat 2.5g	3%
Saturated Fat 1.5g	8%
Trans Fat 0.0g	
Cholesterol 10.0mg	3%
Sodium 75.0mg	3%
Total Carbohydrates 20.0g	7%
Dietary Fiber 0.0g	0%
Total Sugars 18.0g	
Protein 10.0g	20%

* The % Daily Value (DV) tells you how much a nutrient in a serving of food contributes to a daily diet. 2,000 calories a day is used for general nutrition advice.

INGREDIENTS: Cultured Reduced Fat Milk, Water, Cane Sugar, Fruit Puree Blend (Strawberry, Blueberry, Blackberry, Raspberry), Fruit Pectin, Natural Flavors, Fruit and Vegetable Juice Concentrate (for Color), Guar Gum, Lemon Juice Concentrate, Locust Bean Gum, Vanilla Extract, 6 Live and Active Cultures: S. Thermophilus, L. Bulgaricus, L. Acidophilus, Bifidus, L. Casei, and L. Rhamnosus.

Oats

Nutrition Facts

13 servings per container
Serving size: 1/2 cup

Amount per serving
Calories 150

	% Daily Value*
Total Fat 2.5g	3%
Saturated Fat 0.0g	0%
Trans Fat 0.0g	
Cholesterol 0.0mg	0%
Sodium 0.0mg	0%
Total Carbohydrates 27.0g	10%
Dietary Fiber 4.0g	14%
Total Sugars 0.0g	
Protein 5.0g	10%

* The % Daily Value (DV) tells you how much a nutrient in a serving of food contributes to a daily diet. 2,000 calories a day is used for general nutrition advice.

INGREDIENTS: Organic Rolled Oats

Kid's Protein Brownie Bar

Nutrition Facts

1 servings per container
Serving size: 1

Amount per serving
Calories 130

	% Daily Value*
Total Fat 4.0g	5%
Saturated Fat 1.0g	5%
Trans Fat 0.0g	
Cholesterol 0.0mg	0%
Sodium 120.0mg	5%
Total Carbohydrates 25.0g	9%
Dietary Fiber 3.0g	11%
Total Sugars 11.0g	
Protein 2.0g	4%

* The % Daily Value (DV) tells you how much a nutrient in a serving of food contributes to a daily diet. 2,000 calories a day is used for general nutrition advice.

INGREDIENTS: FLOUR, OAT FIBER, TAPIOCA SYRUP, CANE SYRUP, FIG PASTE, CANE SUGAR, COCOA, UNSWEETENED CHOCOLATE, SUNFLOWER AND/OR SOYBEAN OIL, NATURAL FLAVORS, COCOA BUTTER, SALT, BAKING SODA, SOY LECITHIN, VANILLA EXTRACT, MIXED TOCOPHEROLS (ANTIOXIDANT).

Hummus

Nutrition Facts

8 servings per container
Serving size: 2 tablespoon

Amount per serving
Calories 50

	% Daily Value*
Total Fat 2.0g	3%
Saturated Fat 0.0g	0%
Trans Fat 0.0g	
Cholesterol 0.0mg	0%
Sodium 120.0mg	5%
Total Carbohydrates 5.0g	2%
Dietary Fiber 3.0g	11%
Total Sugars 0.0g	
Protein 3.0g	6%

* The % Daily Value (DV) tells you how much a nutrient in a serving of food contributes to a daily diet. 2,000 calories a day is used for general nutrition advice.

INGREDIENTS: Chick Peas, Tahini (Sesame Seeds), Lemon Juice, Garlic, Salt, Citric Acid, Olive Oil

Which 2 foods are the ultra-processed foods?

1.

2.

WORKSHEET 15:
INVESTIGATING INGREDIENT LISTS

1. What are some surprising ingredients you saw on the labels today?

_____
_____
_____
_____
_____
_____

2. Why is it important to know the ingredients in your food?

_____
_____
_____
_____
_____
_____

WORKSHEET 15:
INVESTIGATING INGREDIENT LISTS

3. "I was surprised that _ _ _ _ _ _ _ _ had so many ingredients."

_____
_____
_____
_____
_____
_____
_____
_____

4. "Some real foods I like that only have one ingredient are..."

_____
_____
_____
_____
_____
_____
_____
_____

LESSON 16:

FINDING FAT ON LABELS

> Your brain is made of about 60% fat! But not all fats are equal. Monounsaturated and omega-3 fats help your brain and memory. These healthy fats can be found in nuts, seeds, avocados, some fish (like salmon), and olives. Trans fats and too much saturated fat, found in fast food, packaged food and fried food, can harm your heart and your health.
>
> When looking at labels, it is best to look at the total amount of fat, the amount of trans fat, and the amount of saturated fat. It is best to eat foods that are low in saturated fat and contain no trans fat.
>
> But just looking at the amount of fat does not tell us the full story! In order to determine if you are eating omega-6 fats, omega-3 fats or monounsaturated fats, you will need to look closely at the ingredient list. If you see added oils like sunflower oil, safflower oil, canola oil, vegetable oil, corn oil, or soybean oil, which are found in many ultra-processed foods– you will be eating more omega-6 fats. If the food has ingredients such as nuts, seeds, olives, or avocados, then it contains more of the healthy omega-3 fats or monounsaturated fats.

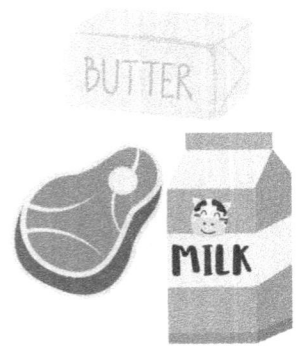

Saturated Fats

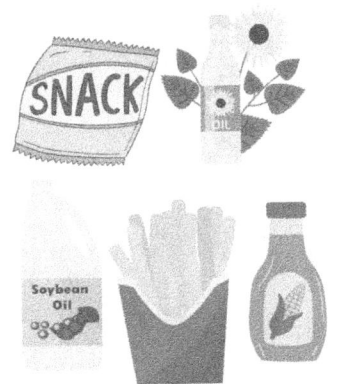

Omega-6 Fats

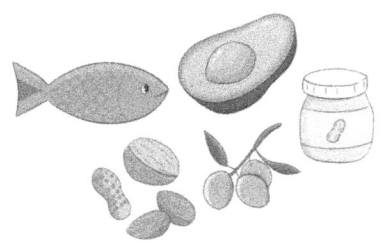

Healthy "Brain Building Fats": Mono-Unsaturated Fats and Omega-3 Fats

WORKSHEET 16:

FINDING FAT ON LABELS

Compare the sample food labels:

<u>Frozen Breakfast sandwich</u> (with egg, sausage, and cheese)

<u>Homemade breakfast sandwich</u> (with Ezekial English Muffin, egg, and avocado)

- Highlight total fat, saturated fat, trans fat.
- Look at the ingredients for added oils and fat.
- Identify which foods contain "brain-building fats" vs "not-so-great fats." Circle the healthy fats. Put an X next to the other "not-so-great fats."

Frozen Breakfast Sandwich

Nutrition Facts

8 servings per container
Serving size: One Sandwich 128 g

Amount per serving
Calories 400

	% Daily Value*
Total Fat 26.0g	33%
Saturated Fat 10.0g	50%
Trans Fat 0.0g	
Cholesterol 120.0mg	40%
Sodium 610.0mg	27%
Total Carbohydrates 29.0g	11%
Dietary Fiber 2.0g	7%
Total Sugars 5.0g	
Protein 13.0g	26%

INGREDIENTS: Croissant: Enriched Bleached Wheat Flour (Contains Bleached Wheat Flour, Malted Barley Flour, Niacin, Reduced Iron, Thiamin Mononitrate, Riboflavin And Folic Acid), Water, Vegetable Oil (Palm, Soybean), High Fructose Corn Syrup, Yeast. Contains 2% Or Less: Isolated Soy Product, Eggs, Salt, Whey, Preservatives (Calcium Propionate, Potassium Sorbate, Sodium Benzoate), Mono And Diglycerides, Maltodextrin, Sugar, Natural And Artificial Flavor, Medium Chain Triglycerides, Soy Lecithin. Fully Cooked Pork and Chicken Sausage Patty: Pork Mechanically Separated Chicken, Water, Soy Protein Concentrate. Contains 2% Or Less: Salt, Pork Stock, Spices, Dextrose, Sodium Phosphates, Sugar, Monosodium Glutamate, Citric Acid, Flavor, Caramel Color. Fully Cooked Egg Patty: Whole Eggs, Nonfat Milk, Soybean Oil, Modified Corn Starch, Salt, Xanthan Gum, Natural And Artificial Butter Flavor (Soybean Oil, Butter, Lipolyzed Butter Oil, And Natural And Artificial Flavors), Citric Acid. Pasteurized Process American Cheese (Milk, Water, Cream. Contains 2% Or Less Of: Cheese Culture, Citric Acid, Color Added, Enzymes, Potassium Citrate, Salt, Sodium Citrate, Sorbic Acid (Preservative), Soy Lecithin, Tetrasodium Pyrophosphate).

Homemade Breakfast Sandwich

Nutrition Facts

Portion Size: 1 Sandwich

Amount Per Portion
Calories 357

	% Daily Value *
Total Fat 17g	22 %
Saturated Fat 2.8g	14 %
Cholesterol 164mg	55 %
Sodium 238mg	10 %
Total Carbohydrate 36g	13 %
Dietary Fiber 11g	39 %
Sugar 0 g	
Protein 17g	34 %
Vitamin D 0.9mcg **	4 %
Calcium 33mg	3 %
Iron 3.3mg	18 %
Potassium 586mg	12 %

Ingredients: Ezekial Sprouted Grain English Muffins (Organic Sprouted Wheat, Organic Sprouted Barley, Organic Sprouted Lentils, Organic Sprouted Soybeans, Organic Sprouted Spelt, Filtered Water, Yeast, Organic Wheat Gluten, Sea Salt), Organic Pasture-Raised Egg, Organic Avocado.

WORKSHEET 16:

FINDING FAT ON LABELS

1. What are some healthy fats you already eat?

----

2. "One way I can help my brain is by eating more..."

----

3. "Next time I choose a snack, I'll check the fat label for..."

LESSON 17:

SLEUTHING SODIUM ON LABELS

> Did you know that large amounts of sodium (salt) are often added to ultra processed foods? While some sodium can make food taste good and last longer, too much sodium is unhealthy for our heart and blood vessels. When we cook food at home and add salt, it is typically a normal amount of sodium. But food manufacturers intentionally add a lot of extra sodium to ultra-processed food, because this helps the food industry make more money. The extra sodium makes people crave more ultra-processed foods.

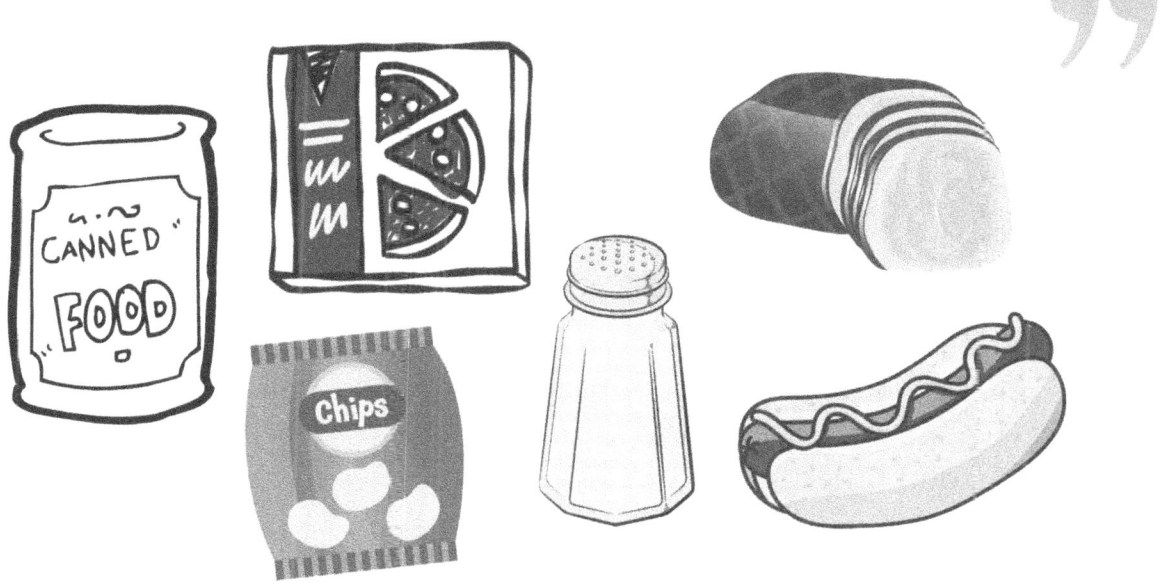

WORKSHEET 17:

SLEUTHING SODIUM ON LABELS

Compare the food labels for homemade pizza vs packaged frozen pizza:

Homemade pizza

Nutrition Facts	
Portion Size	1/3 Pizza
Amount Per Portion	
Calories	**458**
	% Daily Value*
Total Fat 16g	21 %
Saturated Fat 5.6g **	28 %
Cholesterol 32mg **	11 %
Sodium 397mg	17 %
Total Carbohydrate 63g	23 %
Dietary Fiber 6.4g	23 %
Sugar 8.4g	
Protein 21g	42 %
Vitamin D 0.2mcg **	1 %
Calcium 209mg **	16 %
Iron 0.2mg **	1 %
Potassium 395mg	8 %

Ingredients: Organic 100% Whole Wheat Pizza Crust, Organic tomato sauce, Organic Mozzarella Cheese

Frozen pizza

Nutrition Facts	
1 servings per container	
Serving size	2 Slices
Amount per serving	
Calories	**790**
	% Daily Value*
Total Fat 36g	46%
Saturated Fat 17g	85%
Trans Fat 1g	
Cholesterol 90mg	28%
Sodium 1820mg	79%
Total Carbohydrate 82g	30%
Dietary Fiber 5g	18%
Total Sugars 8g	
Includes 4g Added Sugars	8%
Protein 38g	76%
Vitamin D 2mcg	8%
Calcium 680mg	52%
Iron 5mg	29%
Potassium 590mg	13%

INGREDIENTS: Bread (Enriched Wheat Flour [Wheat Flour, Malted Barley Flour, Niacin, Iron, Thiamin Mononitrate, Riboflavin, Folic Acid], Water, Yeast, 2% or Less of Soybean Oil, Wheat Gluten, Salt, Sugar, Acetic Acid, Lactic Acid, Fumaric Acid, Ascorbic Acid, Enzymes, Calcium Propionate [Preservative]), Cheese Mozzarella Part Skim (Pasteurized Part Skim Milk, Cheese Cultures, Salt, Enzymes), Sauce (Water, Tomato Paste, Sugar, Soybean Oil, 2% or Less of Modified Food Starch, Garlic, Spices, Salt, Distilled Vinegar, Onion, Cultured Dextrose, Potassium Chloride, Garlic Powder, Paprika, Natural Hickory Smoke Flavor), Margarine (Soybean Oil, Water, Mono & Diglycerides, 2% or Less of Salt, Natural Flavor, Vitamin A Palmitate, Vitamin D3)

Compare the sodium in the homemade pizza vs the prepackaged pizza. Are you surprised at the difference?

_____

_____

If you are eating a diet of mostly home cooked foods like this, how much sodium would you get in a day? How does that compare with how much sodium is recommended?

_____

_____

If you are eating a diet of mostly prepackaged foods like this, how much sodium would you get in a day? How does that compare with how much sodium is recommended?

_____

_____

WORKSHEET 17:
SLEUTHING SODIUM ON LABELS

1. What kind of foods can you choose for breakfast to avoid eating too much sodium?

_____

_____

_____

_____

2. What kind of foods can you choose for lunch to avoid eating too much sodium?

_____

_____

_____

_____

3. What kind of foods can you choose for dinner to avoid eating too much sodium?

_____

_____

_____

_____

LESSON 18:

UNCOVERING ULTRA-PROCESSED FOODS

"Ultra-processed foods are made in factories, stripped of fiber and nutrients, and often contain ingredients that sound like they were made in a chemistry lab. Most fast food and packaged snacks fall into this category. **When we eat more whole foods, we will automatically have less room on our plates for the ultra-processed ones.**"

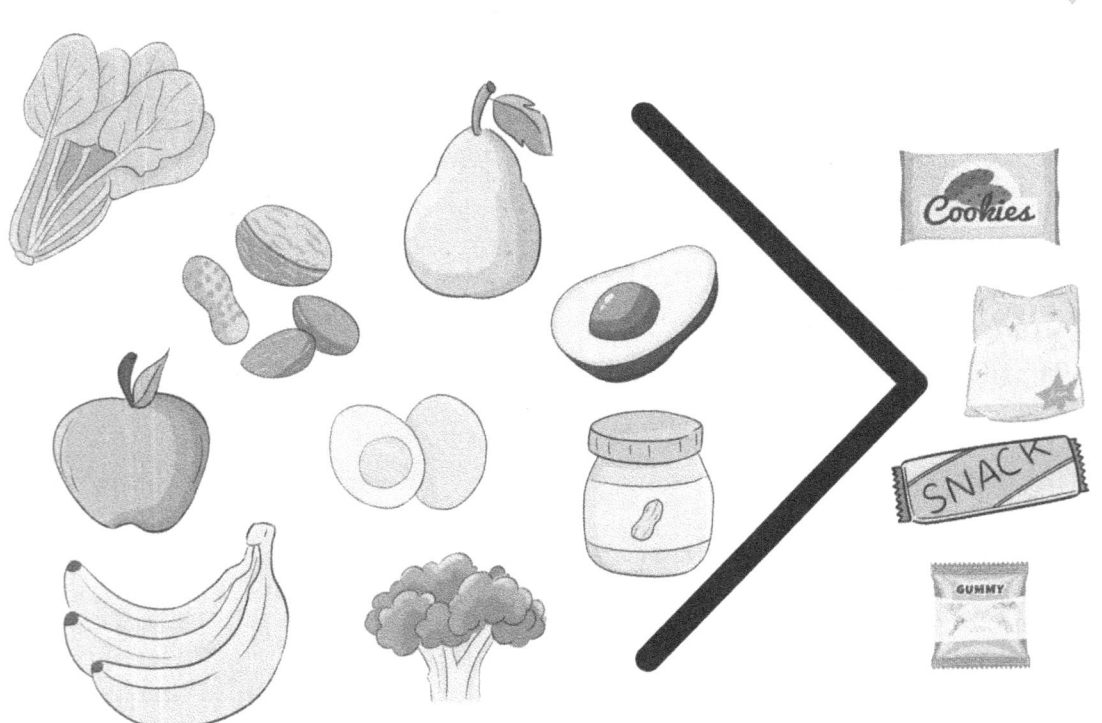

WORKSHEET 18:

UNCOVERING ULTRA-PROCESSED FOODS

Using the labels below, sort each food into the correct category:

Peanut Butter #1
INGREDIENTS: PEANUTS, SALT
CONTAINS: PEANUTS

Peanuts
INGREDIENTS: PEANUTS, SALT
CONTAINS: PEANUTS

Peanut Butter #2
INGREDIENTS: Roasted Peanuts, Sugar, Contains 2% Or Less Of: Molasses, Fully Hydrogenated Vegetable Oils (rapeseed And Soybean), Mono And Diglycerides, Salt.

Apple
INGREDIENTS: ORGANIC APPLE

Apple Sauce #1
INGREDIENTS: Apples, High Fructose Corn Syrup, Water, Ascorbic Acid (Vitamin C).

Apple Sauce #2
INGREDIENTS: ORGANIC APPLES

Popcorn Kernels
INGREDIENTS: ORGANIC POPCORN
MAY CONTAIN MILK AND SOY

Popped Popcorn Snack
INGREDIENTS: ORGANIC NON-GMO POPCORN, ORGANIC EXTRA VIRGIN COCONUT OIL, HIMALAYAN SALT

Cheese Curls Snack
INGREDIENTS: Enriched Corn Meal (Corn Meal, Ferrous Sulfate, Niacin, Thiamin Mononitrate, Riboflavin, Folic Acid), Vegetable Oil (Corn, Canola, and/or Sunflower Oil), Cheese Seasoning (Whey, Cheddar Cheese [Milk, Cheese Cultures, Salt, Enzymes], Canola Oil, Maltodextrin [Made from Corn], Natural and Artificial Flavors, Salt, Whey Protein Concentrate, Monosodium Glutamate, Lactic Acid, Citric Acid, Artificial Color [Yellow 6]), and Salt.

Whole Food	Lightly Processed	Ultra-Processed

WORKSHEET 18:
UNCOVERING ULTRA-PROCESSED FOODS

1. What clues helped you know a food was ultra-processed?

_____

_____

_____

_____

_____

_____

_____

_____

2. What are some examples of ingredients you saw in the ultra-processed foods, that you did not see in the lightly processed foods?

_____

_____

_____

_____

_____

_____

_____

WORKSHEET 18:
UNCOVERING ULTRA-PROCESSED FOODS

3. "Some ultra-processed foods I used to eat often were..."

_____
_____
_____
_____
_____
_____
_____
_____
_____
_____

4. "Now I want to try eating more _____ instead."

_____
_____
_____
_____
_____
_____
_____
_____
_____

LESSON 19:

FOODS PRETENDING TO BE HEALTHY WITH A HEALTH HALO

"Some foods are marketed to look healthy, like granola bars or veggie chips—but many of them are ultra-processed and full of added sugars, unhealthy fats, or artificial ingredients. That's the health halo effect!

A halo is a glowing circle you sometimes see drawn around people's heads in cartoons or pictures to show that they're good. The health halo is when a food seems healthy—because of the way it's packaged, labeled, or advertised—even if it's not the best choice.

For example, if a snack says "low fat," "natural," or "gluten-free," some people might think it's super healthy—without actually looking at what's really inside. But guess what? That same snack might still be full of sugar, artificial ingredients, or barely any nutrients at all.

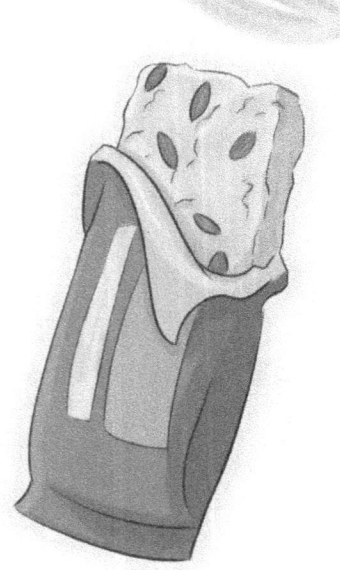

The best way to know if something is actually healthy is to look closely at the ingredients and ask:
Is this a whole food? Is it full of good stuff like fiber or nutrients? Or does this have lots of ultra-processed ingredients like sugar, salt, or added oils?"

WORKSHEET 19:

FOODS PRETENDING TO BE HEALTHY WITH A HEALTH HALO

Look around your pantry, fridge, or in the grocery store and find four foods with a "health halo". List the product names and describe their "health halos".

Product Name	Health Halo Description
Example: Dark Chocolate Cocoa Protein Bar	On the package it says, "good source of protein," "made with super grains," "gluten free," and "100% whole grains." The packaging makes it look really natural and healthy. But, when I look at the label, there are lots of ingredients that I wouldn't find in a normal kitchen, like added oils and added sugar-- I can tell it's an ultra-processed food. It also has 9 grams of added sugar! A better choice would be some homemade trail mix or nuts for a high protein snack.

WORKSHEET 19:

FOODS PRETENDING TO BE HEALTHY WITH A HEALTH HALO

1. Why do some snacks sound healthier than they really are?

----

2. What are foods you used to think were healthy but now know aren't?

----

3. "Some whole foods I can eat instead are…"

LESSON 20:

CREATING AN INCREDIBLE PLATE

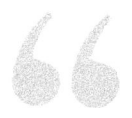

In order to get all of the nutrients you need, it is important to include all of the food groups.

Here is what we can aim for:

1. **For every meal, try to make half of your plate fruits and vegetables!** Choose a variety of vegetables and whole fruits with lots of different colors! By doing this, we will be eating lots of fiber, micronutrients, phytonutrients, and healthy carbohydrates.

2. **For every meal, make one quarter of your plate healthy protein.** The healthiest sources of protein are plant proteins (like beans, lentils, nuts, and seeds), pasture-raised eggs, fish, and lean meats like chicken breast. Aim to eat these healthier sources of protein in place of red meat and processed meats (ex. hot dogs and sausage) which are not as healthy for your body. Eating protein at every meal is important because when we eat enough protein, we are giving our bodies what they need to build new cells and build muscle.

3. **Make one quarter of your plate whole grains.** This includes foods like oats, brown rice, whole grain pasta, quinoa, and whole wheat bread, rather than white rice, white pasta, or white bread. Eating whole grains is important, because whole grains are a healthy source of complex carbohydrates that will give us sustained energy. Whole grains will also provide nutrients and fiber for our microbiome.

4. **Include healthy fats to your diet every day**. Examples are foods like nuts, seeds, olives, fish, or avocados. This is important because healthy fats are important for our cell and brain health.

5. **Drink water**, as the drink of choice with every meal or snack, rather than drinking juice or sugary beverages. Water is the best choice for quenching our thirst.

6. **Try to include some foods on your plate every day that are a good source of calcium.** Green leafy vegetables (ex. kale), almonds, chia seeds, tofu, and fortified soy milk are great non-dairy options. Dairy products including milk, yogurt, and cheese are good sources of calcium.

LESSON 20:

CREATING AN INCREDIBLE PLATE

For every meal (breakfast, lunch, and dinner), try to aim for your plate to look like this.

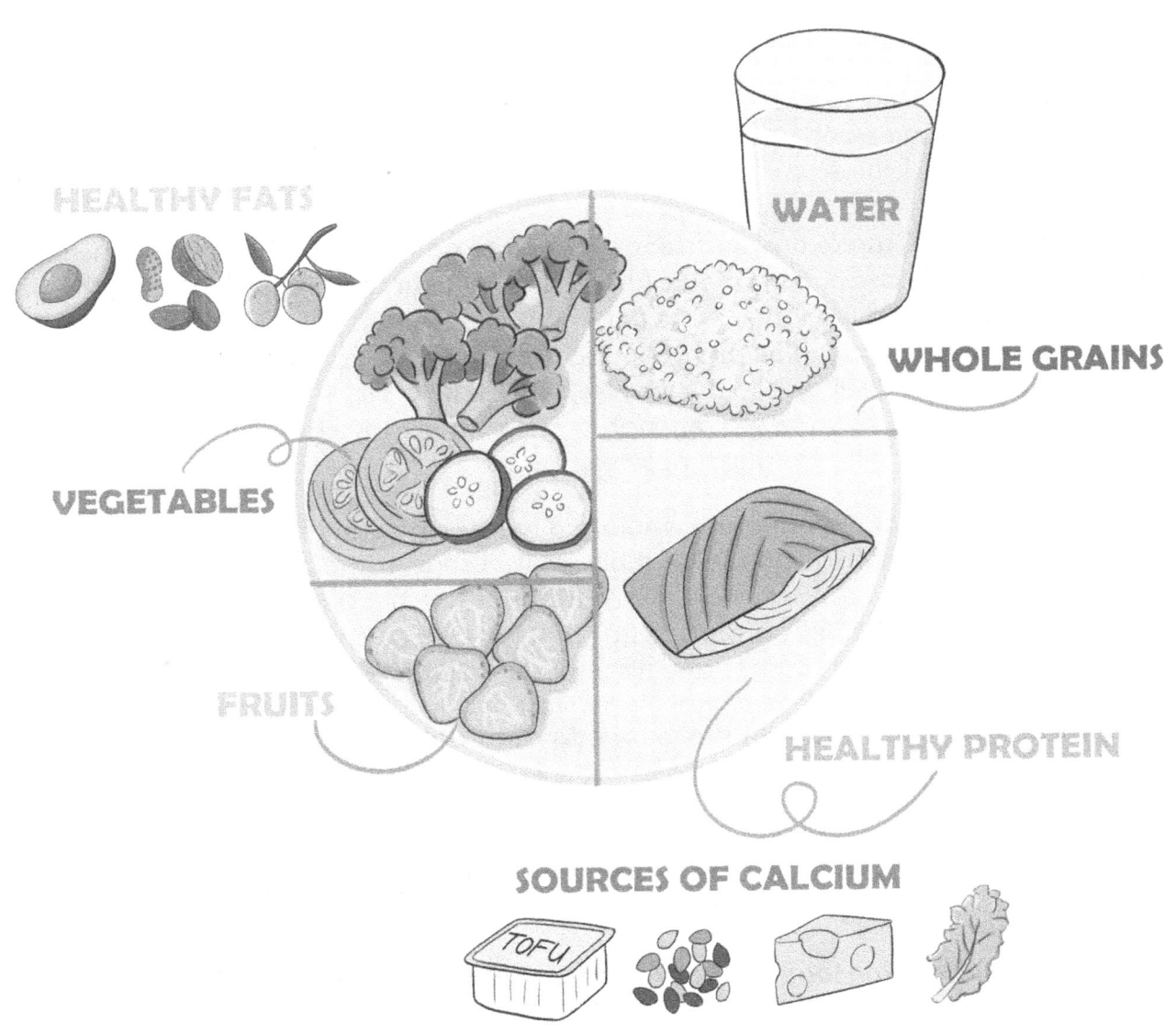

WORKSHEET 20:

CREATING AN INCREDIBLE PLATE

Create a few plates of your own for breakfast, lunch and dinner. Try to include all of the components shown on the sample plate: fruits and veggies, healthy proteins, and whole grains. Try to include some healthy fats. Then describe the plate, explaining why it's a balanced meal.

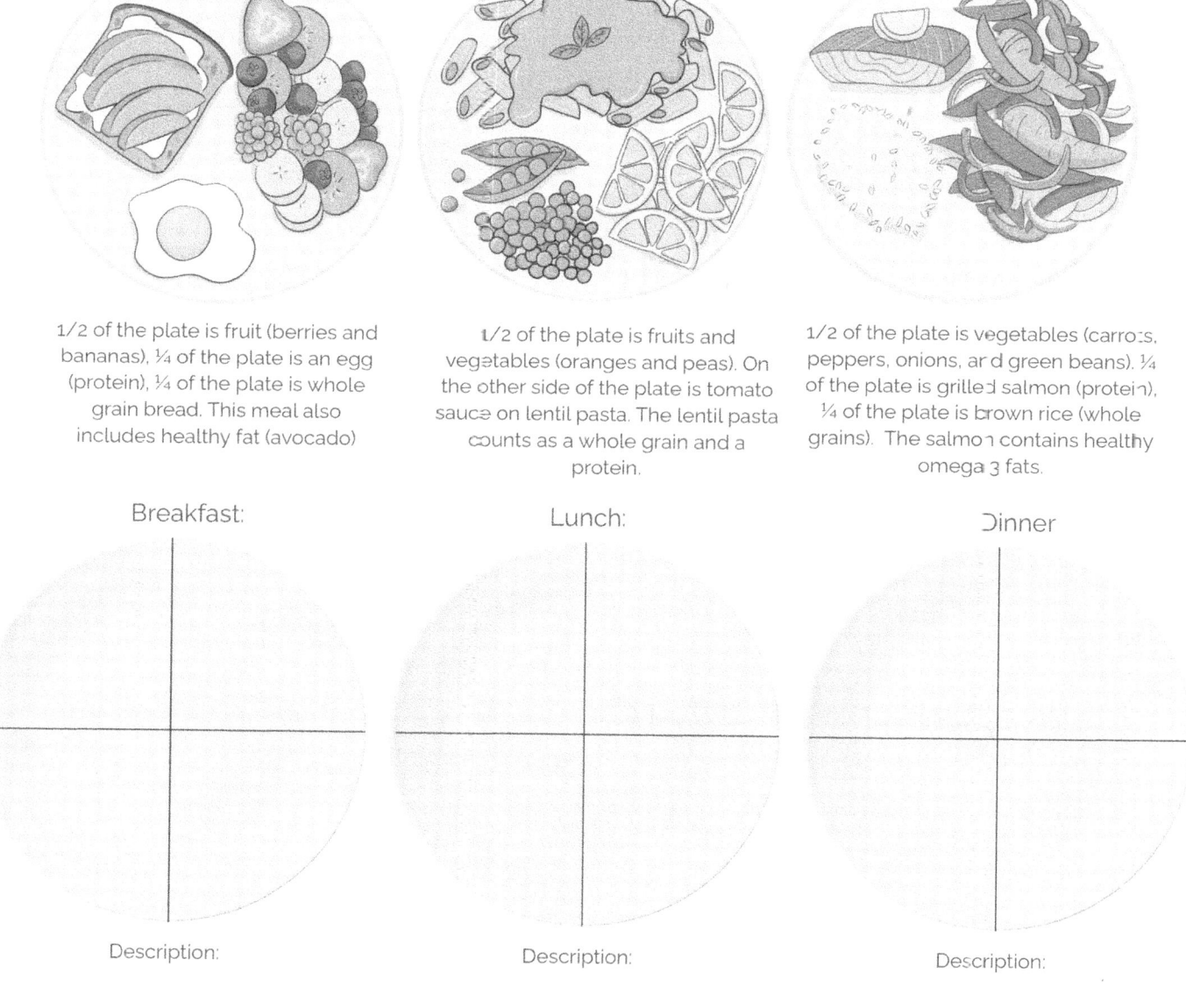

Sample Breakfast:

1/2 of the plate is fruit (berries and bananas), ¼ of the plate is an egg (protein), ¼ of the plate is whole grain bread. This meal also includes healthy fat (avocado)

Sample Lunch:

1/2 of the plate is fruits and vegetables (oranges and peas). On the other side of the plate is tomato sauce on lentil pasta. The lentil pasta counts as a whole grain and a protein.

Sample Dinner:

1/2 of the plate is vegetables (carrots, peppers, onions, and green beans). ¼ of the plate is grilled salmon (protein), ¼ of the plate is brown rice (whole grains). The salmon contains healthy omega 3 fats.

Breakfast:

Description:

Lunch:

Description:

Dinner

Description:

WORKSHEET 20:

CREATING AN INCREDIBLE PLATE

1. Why is it important to have a balanced plate for every meal (breakfast, lunch and dinner)?

---

2. Some of the food groups that I want to eat more of are...

---

3. What are some foods you can add to your plate, to make your breakfast, lunch, and dinner more balanced?

LESSON 21:
THE POWER OF PROTEIN FROM PLANTS

> "Beans, lentils, tofu, nuts, and seeds are all amazing sources of plant-based protein. These foods also contain fiber, micronutrients, and healthy fats. And they're healthy for your body and the planet!"

SOURCES OF PLANT PROTEIN

100g **TEMPEH**	1 cup cooked **LENTILS**	2 tbsp **PEANUT BUTTER**	1 cup **STEAMED KALE**
18 g Protein	18 g Protein	8 g Protein	3 g Protein

½ cup shelled **EDAMAME** 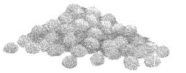	1 cup cooked **KIDNEY BEANS** 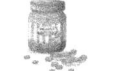	1 cup cooked **Quinoa** 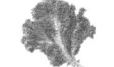	½ cup **ROLLED OATS**
13 g Protein	13 g Protein	8 g Protein	5 g Protein

100g **FIRM TOFU** 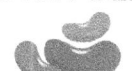	1 cup cooked **CHICKPEAS** 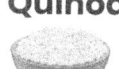	2 Tbsp **NUTRITIONAL YEAST** 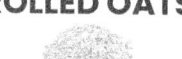	3 Tbsp **HEMP SEEDS** 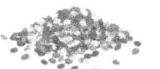
12 g Protein	12 g Protein	12 g Protein	10 g Protein

WORKSHEET 21:

THE POWER OF PROTEIN FROM PLANTS

1. Did anything surprise you about how much protein is in plants?

_____
_____
_____
_____
_____
_____
_____

2. What plant proteins would you like to try?

_____
_____
_____
_____
_____
_____
_____

WORKSHEET 21:
THE POWER OF PROTEIN FROM PLANTS

3. "Today I learned that _____ are great protein sources!"

_____
_____
_____
_____
_____
_____
_____
_____

4. "Some plant based meals I want to try making are..."

_____
_____
_____
_____
_____
_____
_____
_____

LESSON 22:

NOURISH YOUR BODY AND HEAL THE EARTH

> Eating more plants and whole foods is healthier for you, but it also helps the Earth. Plants take less energy, water, and land to produce than animal products. Ultra-processed foods often come in plastic packages, use more fossil fuels, and create more pollution than whole foods. Choosing whole foods that are local and organic, when possible, is even better!

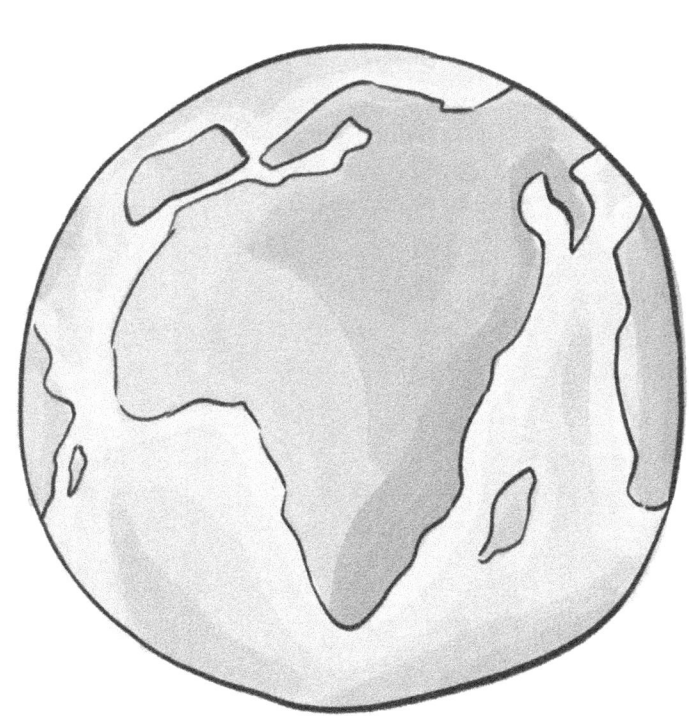

WORKSHEET 22:

NOURISH YOUR BODY AND HEAL THE EARTH

Compare the two foods and determine which is "Better for the Earth" vs. "Not as Earth-Friendly."

- **Circle the food that is Better for the Earth.**

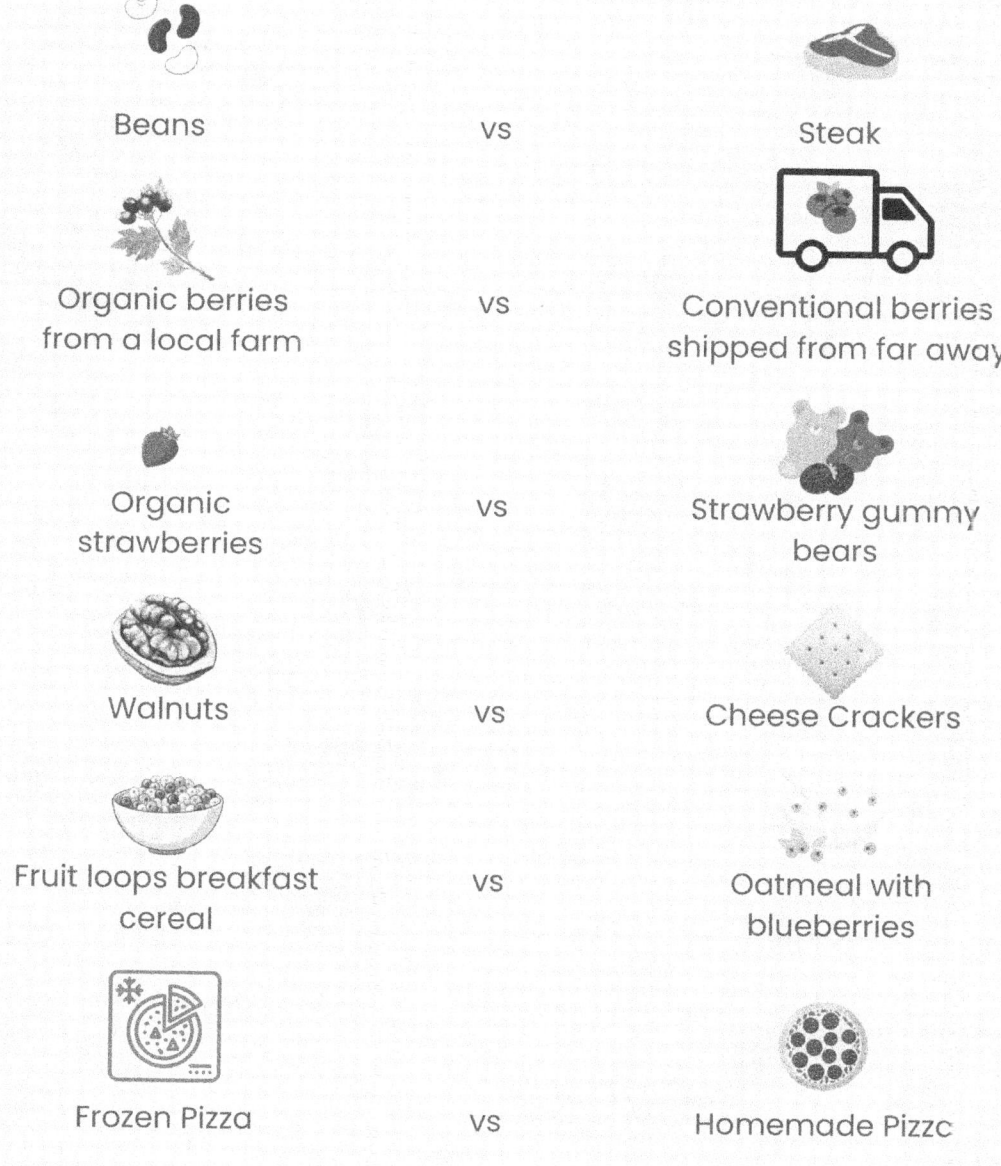

Beans	vs	Steak
Organic berries from a local farm	vs	Conventional berries shipped from far away
Organic strawberries	vs	Strawberry gummy bears
Walnuts	vs	Cheese Crackers
Fruit loops breakfast cereal	vs	Oatmeal with blueberries
Frozen Pizza	vs	Homemade Pizza

- **Now put a star by the foods that are healthier for you.**

WORKSHEET 22:

NOURISH YOUR BODY AND HEAL THE EARTH

1. What are 3 Earth-friendly foods you have eaten recently?

    1. _____
    2. _____
    3. _____

2. What are some swaps you can make to eat more Earth-friendly foods?

    1. _____
    2. _____
    3. _____

3. Why should we be concerned about the health of the planet?

    _____
    _____
    _____
    _____
    _____

WORKSHEET 22:

NOURISH YOUR BODY AND HEAL THE EARTH

1. Why are the foods that are healthier for the planet also healthier for your health?

----

2. How does your plate affect the planet?

----

3. What are some changes you could make to your plate that would make a big difference for Earth?

LESSON 23:

THE MEDIA AND OUR HEALTH

> Have you ever wondered why certain foods are advertised more often than others? Who helps you decide what to eat? Do you ever see food ads on TV or the internet? Do you ever hear about foods that are popular or trendy? What do they try to make you feel or believe?
>
> It seems like everywhere we look, there are messages telling us what to buy, what to eat, and what is healthy. But how do we know who to trust? A lot of these messages come from food companies who want to sell their products, or diet companies who want to sell their programs.

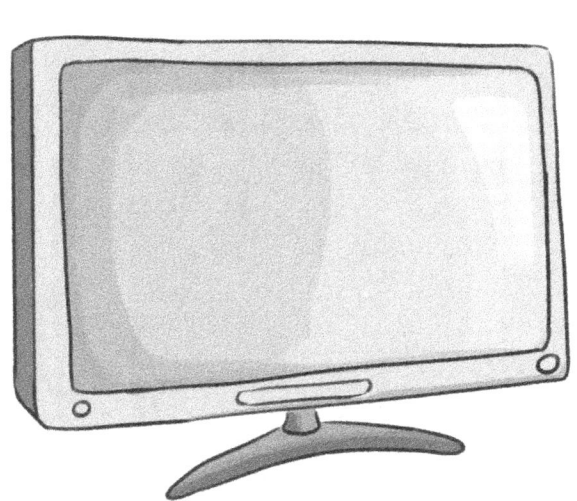

WORKSHEET 23:

THE MEDIA AND OUR HEALTH

Think about some of the food advertisements and food trends you have seen. List 3 media influences that may have affected you:

1.
2.
3.

1. What foods were they selling? Were the advertisements for whole foods or ultra-processed foods?
_____
_____
_____

2. What were they trying to make you feel or believe?
_____
_____
_____

3. What did they say or show to make the foods seem appealing?
_____
_____
_____

4. How did the advertisements make you feel? Did they make you want to try the foods?
_____
_____

WORKSHEET 23:

THE MEDIA AND OUR HEALTH

1. Why is it important to notice the forces that influence our choices?

_____
_____
_____
_____

2. Why might food manufacturers spend lots of money to create advertisements?

_____
_____
_____
_____

3. What are some places we can find information we can trust?

_____
_____
_____
_____

LESSON 24:

MY WEEKLY WINS!

> We don't have to be perfect, but every time we eat, we have a chance to make a powerful choice. When we eat food that gives us good energy and sends healthy messages to our body, we are taking care of ourselves—and that's something to feel proud of.
>
> If we can increase the amount of whole foods that we are eating while we reduce the amount of ultra-processed food that we are eating, this is a great first step!
>
> Rather than focusing on **cutting out** the ultra-processed foods, a better approach is to focus on **crowding out** the ultra-processed foods.
>
> **Crowding out means, if you focus on trying to eat more or mostly whole foods, you will naturally have less room on your plate and in your stomach for the processed foods. Similarly, when you choose to eat something processed, if you try to choose more slightly processed foods, you will have less room on your plate for the ultra-processed foods.**

Use the "My Weekly Wins" worksheet to help you feel good about making healthy choices! This week, color in a star every time you eat these healthy foods, or do these healthy habits! How many "wins" can you get this week?

WORKSHEET 24:
MY WEEKLY WINS!

My Weekly Wins
Color in a star whenever you eat these foods or do these things!

fruits ☆☆☆☆☆

tomatoes or tomato sauce ☆☆☆☆☆

be kind to someone ☆☆☆☆☆

berries ☆☆☆☆☆

legumes (beans or lentils) ☆☆☆☆☆

run, swim or play a sport ☆☆☆☆☆

garden veggies ☆☆☆☆☆

nuts and seeds ☆☆☆☆☆

play outside ☆☆☆☆☆

Powerhouse veggies ☆☆☆☆☆

get enough sleep ☆☆☆☆☆

drink water ☆☆☆☆☆

whole grains ☆☆☆☆☆

think of something you are grateful for ☆☆☆☆☆

Have fun! ☆☆☆☆☆

How many wins can you get this week?

WORKSHEET 24:

MY WEEKLY WINS!

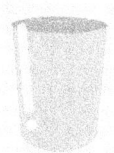

Drink Water. Water makes up 60% of our bodies! Water helps our bodies do the things it needs to do to stay healthy. When you are thirsty, water is the best choice!

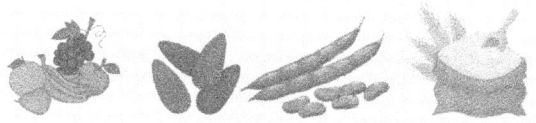

Fruits, Vegetables, Beans, Nuts, Seeds, and Whole Grains all have lots of important nutrients as well as fiber. It's important to eat a variety of foods because each of them has different nutrients that help keep our bodies functioning well!

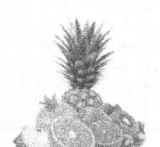

Fruits. Apples, oranges, bananas, grapes, pineapple, mango, peaches, and pears are some examples of fruits... and did you know avocados are a fruit, too?

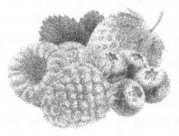

Berries. Although berries are a kind of fruit, they get their own category because they are filled with antioxidants, which are special substances that protect our cells. They also have a lot of fiber, even though they are small.

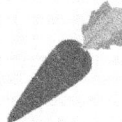

Garden Vegetables. Cucumbers, Carrots, Peppers, Celery, Zucchini, and Squash are just a few examples of vegetables that are full of fiber, vitamins and minerals.

Tomatoes. Tomatoes are officially a fruit but they get their own category because they contain a very important antioxidant known as lycopene which helps our hearts. Did you know that tomato sauce is super healthy too?

WORKSHEET 24:

MY WEEKLY WINS!

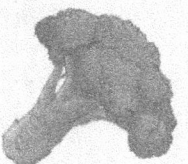

Powerhouse Vegetables. These are also known as cruciferous vegetables and they are packed with important nutrients. These include broccoli, cabbage, cauliflower, brussels sprouts, and some leafy greens like kale and bok choy.

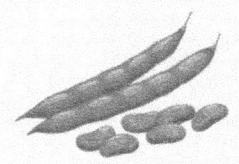

Beans. Beans are full of fiber and nutrients but they also are a great source of plant protein. Plant-based protein is good for everyone, not just vegetarians. Beans are great in burritos and salads and even on their own. Chickpeas (also known as garbanzo beans) are delicious and can be eaten whole or mashed into hummus!

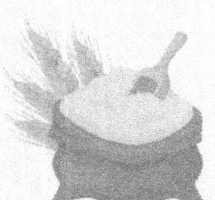

Whole grains. A whole grain is a grain that has all its parts and hasn't been processed to remove the healthy components (the bran, germ, and endosperm). Plain white bread is made with just the endosperm but the bran and germ contain all the healthy parts of the grain! Oats in oatmeal, quinoa, and 100% whole grain bread are all examples of whole grains.

Nuts, Seeds, and nut/seed butter
Nuts and seeds contain protein, fiber, and healthy fats! They can be eaten whole or in nut butter like peanut butter and almond butter. If you are allergic to nuts, then try seed butter. Just remember to choose one without added sugars and when possible, no added oils. The best choices are the ones with the fewest ingredients.

WORKSHEET 24:

MY WEEKLY WINS!

1. Why is it more fun to focus on adding more healthy foods to our plate ("crowding out"), rather than trying to "cut out" foods?

_____
_____
_____
_____
_____
_____
_____
_____

2. How can eating more whole foods and plants help you?

_____
_____
_____
_____
_____
_____
_____
_____

WORKSHEET 24:
MY WEEKLY WINS!

3. "This week I felt proud when I..."

_____
_____
_____
_____
_____
_____
_____

4. Next week, I want to try to eat more of these foods and do more of these things...

_____
_____
_____
_____
_____
_____
_____

LESSON 25:

SHARE WHAT YOU LEARNED!

"

Lots of adults were never taught about food, but you have the power to share what you know! When we talk to our families and friends kindly and confidently, we can help others learn about the power of food and make healthy choices too—without judging or pressuring anyone.

Want to tell someone about what you learned- but not sure how?

Here are some tips to help you talk about food and nutrition with your friends and family:

Be curious, not bossy.
Instead of saying, "You shouldn't eat that!", try saying, "Did you know I learned something cool about food today?"

Share what excites you.
"I just found out how our food can help our brains! Isn't that cool?"

Ask questions.
"What's your favorite fruit or veggie?"

Be kind, even if people don't agree.
It's okay if others make different choices. Your job is to share, not to judge.
When you speak with kindness and excitement, people are more likely to listen!

"

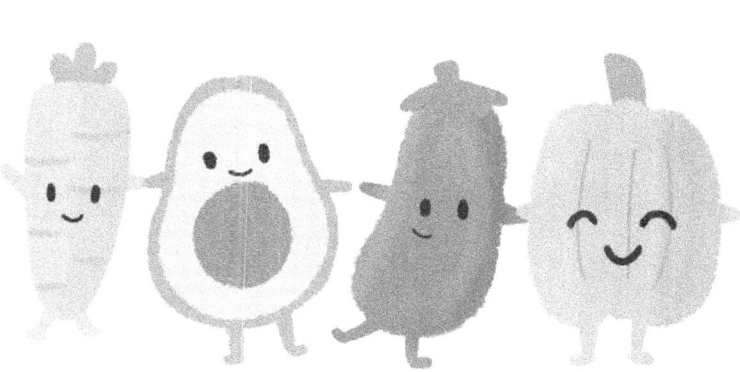

WORKSHEET 25:

SHARE WHAT YOU LEARNED!

Identify 3 people with whom you can share your knowledge from this book.

1. _____
2. _____
3. _____

Using the tips above, write down 3 things you learned that you can share with them, while being kind and curious.

1. _____
_____
_____
_____

2. _____
_____
_____
_____

3. _____
_____
_____
_____

WORKSHEET 25:

SHARE WHAT YOU LEARNED!

1. Why is it important to talk kindly about food?

_____
_____
_____
_____

2. How can you help your family or friends feel curious about food and nutrition—not judged?

_____
_____
_____
_____

3. "Something I want to teach my family is…"

_____
_____
_____
_____

LESSON 26:

MAKING DECISIONS

> Every food we eat sends a message to our body. Some foods help us feel focused, energized, and calm. Others might give us a quick burst, but then make us feel sluggish. When we stop and think about how food makes us feel, we can make better choices—even when tempting options are around.

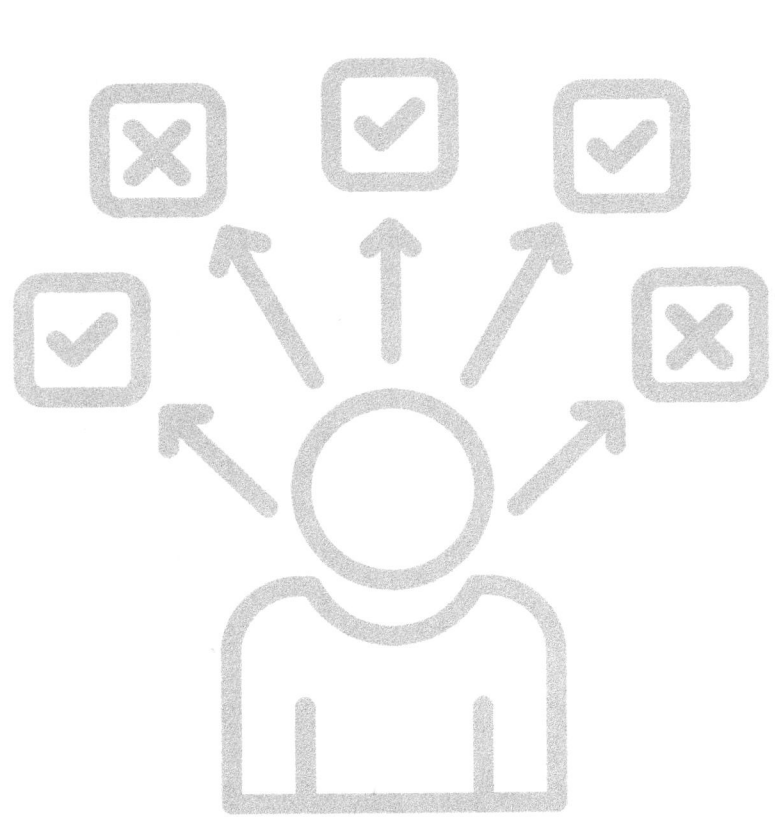

WORKSHEET 26:

MAKING DECISIONS

List 3 snack options, list their ingredients, write how you will feel if you will eat the snack.

Snack	Ingredients	How you feel

▷ Look at three snack options in your kitchen.

▷ Look closely at their labels and write down their ingredients.

▷ Compare the snack options.

▷ Write down how you think they would make you feel.

▷ Put a star on the snack option that is the healthiest.

▷ Circle which snack option you would choose.

WORKSHEET 26:

MAKING DECISIONS

1. Why is it important to look at the label and think about how a food will make you feel, before choosing it?

_____
_____
_____
_____

2. "Some snacks that help me feel great are..."

_____
_____
_____
_____

3. "I feel better when I choose..."

_____
_____
_____
_____

LESSON 27:

SETTING A SMART GOAL

What is a SMART Goal?

SMART stands for:
Specific: Clearly define what you want to accomplish.
Measurable: Make sure you can track your progress.
Achievable: Your goal should be realistic and attainable.
Relevant: It should be important to you and align with your values.
Time-bound: Set a deadline to keep yourself motivated.

For example, setting a goal like, "I want to eat more vegetables", is not specific or time-bound. On the other hand, setting a goal like, "I want half of my plate to be fruits and vegetables for every dinner this week," is specific, measurable, achievable, relevant, and time bound.

Setting SMART goals can help you to be more successful with achieving your goals, because it helps you break down big goals into manageable, specific steps!

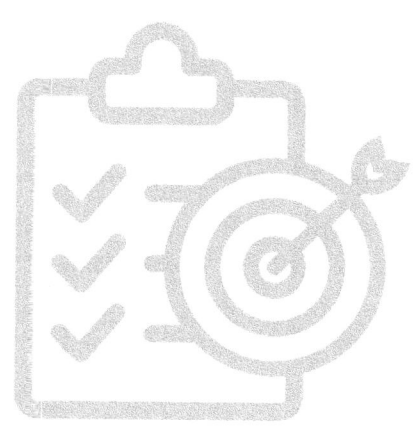

WORKSHEET 27:
SETTING A SMART GOAL

Create your own SMART goal about your nutrition, using these questions to guide you.

SMART Step	My Goal	Question to Think About
Specific	What exactly do I want to achieve?	What do I want to accomplish?
Measurable	How will I know I'm making progress?	How can I track my success?
Achievable	Is this goal realistic for me right now?	Do I have the time and resources to do this?
Relevant	Why is this goal important to me?	How will achieving this help me?
Time-bound	When do I want to complete this goal by?	What is my deadline?

Here is my SMART goal about my nutrition:

WORKSHEET 27:

SETTING A SMART GOAL

1. Why is it important to create SMART goals rather than non-specific goals?

---

2. What are some more SMART goals you want to set regarding your nutrition?

---

3. I am excited to reach my goals because...

LESSON 28:

RECOGNIZING VALID & RELIABLE RESOURCES

> Many adults and kids choose food based on ads or packaging, without realizing that companies are trying to sell us something—often ultra-processed foods. These companies use bright colors, fun characters, and tempting words like 'natural' or 'healthy' to make us think it's a better choice than it really is. When we are deciding if we can trust this information, here are some questions we can ask ourselves:
>
> Who created this?
> Are they trying to sell me something?
> Does this sound science-based?

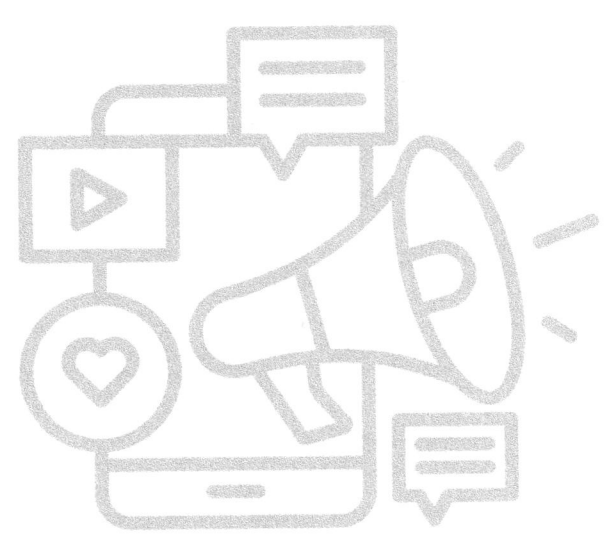

WORKSHEET 28:
RECOGNIZING VALID & RELIABLE RESOURCES

Circle which sources are a valid source to get nutrition information.

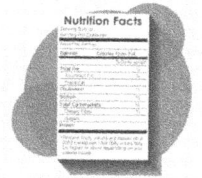
Food Labels

Science Books

Social Media

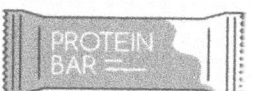
Food trends

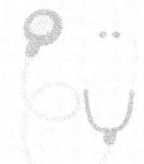
Your Doctor

Television Ads

Online Videos (ex. YouTube and Tiktok)

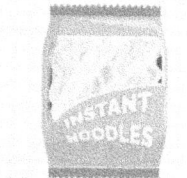
Front of food package

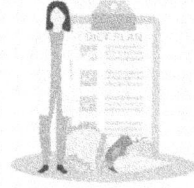
A Nutritionist

Friends

WORKSHEET 28:
RECOGNIZING VALID & RELIABLE RESOURCES

1. Have you ever wanted to try a food just because of an ad?

   _____
   _____
   _____
   _____

2. What can you do to think for yourself when making food choices?

   _____
   _____
   _____
   _____

3. "Next time I see a food ad, I'll remember..."

   _____
   _____
   _____
   _____

WORKSHEET 28:
RECOGNIZING VALID & RELIABLE RESOURCES

4. Why is it important to get your information from reliable sources?

_____
_____
_____
_____
_____
_____
_____
_____

5. What's something you believed before about food/nutrition that turned out not to be true?

_____
_____
_____
_____
_____
_____
_____
_____

WORKSHEET 28:
RECOGNIZING VALID & RELIABLE RESOURCES

6. "Next time I look something up, I'll..."

_____
_____
_____
_____
_____
_____
_____
_____

7. "Some resources I can trust are..."

_____
_____
_____
_____
_____
_____
_____
_____

LESSON 29:

HELPING YOURSELF, HELPING OTHERS, AND HELPING THE EARTH

"You have the power to take care of your body and the Earth. Your voice matters. The food you eat matters. And our world is better when you understand the wonder of what we eat."

WORKSHEET 29:

HELPING YOURSELF, HELPING OTHERS, AND HELPING THE EARTH

Create an Advocacy Letter or a Poster!

- Speak Up for Healthy Choices! Perhaps write a short letter to your school cafeteria suggesting one healthier meal option. Or perhaps make a sign about how the food you eat affects the health of our Earth!

- Include a drawing, fact, or message, from something that you learned.

- Plan your letter or poster here.

- Share your creation with a family member, your teacher, or your friends.

WORKSHEET 29:

HELPING YOURSELF, HELPING OTHERS, AND HELPING THE EARTH

1. Why does your voice matter?

   ----

2. Why is it important to speak up about healthy food choices?

   ----

3. "I'm proud that I..."

LESSON 30:
NEXT STOP– THE GROCERY SHOP!

"So now that you know the truth, what will you choose?

Will you choose foods that help your body feel energized, focused, and strong? Will you choose foods that help your microbiome thrive and your brain feel calm and happy? Will you choose foods that send good messages to your genes, so you stay healthy for years to come? Will you choose foods that protect our Earth, our animals, our soil, our water, and our future?

You don't have to be perfect. But every time you eat, you have a chance to make a powerful choice.

You have the power to take care of your body. You have the power to take care of our Earth.
That power begins with what you put on your plate."

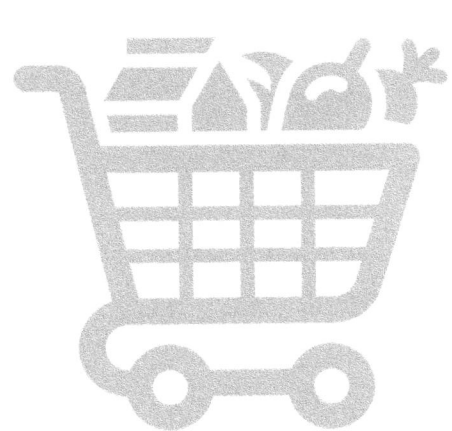

WORKSHEET 30:

NEXT STOP– THE GROCERY SHOP!

Here are some ideas of foods to add to your grocery list...

VEGETABLES:

- Broccoli
- Kale
- Carrots
- Soup starters: Celery, Onions, Garlic, Ginger
- Spinach
- Cauliflower
- Bell Peppers
- Salad add ins: Snap Peas, Beets

FRUITS:

- Berries (ex Blueberries, Raspberries, Strawberries)
- Fruit for snacking: (ex Apples, Oranges, Cherries)
- Lemons, Limes
- Avocados
- Frozen fruit for smoothies (ex. Blueberries, Raspberries, Blackberries, Strawberries)

NUTS, SEEDS, AND NUT BUTTERS:

- Variety of Nuts (ex. Almonds, Cashews, Pistachios, Walnuts, Pecans)
- Nut or seed butters (ex. Peanut butter, Almond Butter, Sunflower Butter)
- Variety of Seeds (ex. Sunflower Seeds, Pumpkin Seeds, Chia Seeds, Flax Seeds, Hemp Seeds)

PLANT BASED PROTEINS:

- Variety of Beans (ex. Black Beans, Chick Peas, Kidney Beans, Cannellini Beans, etc)
- Variety of Lentils (Red, Brown, Black, etc)
- Organic Tofu (Extra Firm for stir fry. Silken for most desserts)
- Peas, Edamame

DAIRY, NON DAIRY MILK AND YOGURT

- Organic Milk (Grass Fed Dairy, or Non-Dairy: ex. Soy Milk)
- Organic Yogurt: Unsweetened, (Grass-Fed Dairy, or Non-Dairy)

ANIMAL BASED PROTEIN (OPTIONAL)

- Salmon (Wild Caught)
- Tuna (Skipjack-Pole and Line Caught)
- Organic Chicken Breast
- Organic Pasture-Raised Eggs

FREQUENTLY ASKED QUESTIONS:

Do I need to follow this list exactly?
NO, this sample grocery list just has some initial suggestions to get you started eating more whole foods and plants. Use the next page to make your own grocery list!

Should I Buy Organic?
USDA certified organic produce is grown without pesticides, fertilizers, or synthetic additives, and is not genetically modified. Animals raised on organic farms are not given antibiotics or growth hormones. For these reasons (and more), when possible, it is better to choose organic over conventional. Buying organic is especially important for: Oats, Whole Wheat, Soy (tofu and soy milk), Corn, Strawberries, Spinach/Greens, Peaches, Pears, Nectarines, Apples, Grapes, Peppers, Cherries, Blueberries, Beans, and all Animal products (meat and dairy).

WORKSHEET 30:

NEXT STOP— THE GROCERY SHOP!

Using everything you have learned, create a grocery list with a parent or family member. What do you want to eat? What do you want to cook? The more incredible foods you have at home, the more likely you will be to eat them! Use the sample grocery list as a guide, and think about which foods you want to eat!

Need some inspiration with easy meal ideas? Want to learn how to cook simple, healthy, and kid-approved recipes for breakfast, lunch, dinner, snack and dessert? Check out "The Wonder of What We Eat Cookbook!"

Make your list, and head to the grocery store!

VEGETABLES	FRUITS	NUTS, SEEDS, AND NUT BUTTERS

PLANT BASED PROTEIN	DAIRY, NON DAIRY MILK AND YOGURT	ANIMAL BASED PROTEIN (OPTIONAL)

WORKSHEET 30:

NEXT STOP— THE GROCERY SHOP!

1. Some foods I want to eat this week for breakfast are…

---

2. Some foods I want to eat this week for lunch are…

---

3. Some foods I want to eat this week for dinner are…

WORKSHEET 30:

NEXT STOP– THE GROCERY SHOP!

4. Learning to cook is one of the best skills you can have, because it lets you choose what goes into your food, so you can have more power over your health.

When you know how to cook, you have the power to take care of yourself, to make yummy meals for the people you love, and to turn simple ingredients into something amazing!

Some foods I want to learn how to cook are...

ANSWER KEY

WORKSHEET 2

Match each part with foods from nature that help it work well:

1. **HEART** — B. Pumps blood and oxygen to your entire body—over 100,000 beats a day!
2. **BRAIN** — A. Sends lightning-fast messages to help you move, think, feel, and remember.
3. **MUSCLES** — D. Power every move you make—from jumping to chewing—over 600 in your body!
4. **LUNGS** — C. Breathe in oxygen and get rid of carbon dioxide—about 20,000 breaths a day!
5. **STOMACH & INTESTINES** — G. Break down food, absorb nutrients, and give you the energy to run, think, and play.
6. **CELLS** — E. Tiny building blocks—trillions of them! They help you grow, heal, and stay strong.
7. **NERVE** — F. Carry messages at over 250 mph from your brain to your body (and back)!

WORKSHEET 3

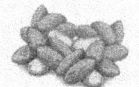 VS

e.g. 1 oz almonds (about 23 almonds) — 160 Kcal
1 oz potato chips (about 20 chips) — 160 Kcal

- ✓ WHICH HAS MORE FIBER?
- ✓ WHICH HAS MORE VITAMINS AND MINERALS?
- ✓ WHICH IS BETTER FOR YOUR MICROBIOME?
- ✓ WHICH WILL GIVE BETTER, LASTING ENERGY?

WORKSHEET 4

List the foods into the correct columns:
(Hint: Some foods can be in more than one column).

Foods:	Carbohydrates	Protein	Healthy Fat
Oatmeal	Oatmeal	Nuts	Nuts
Bananas	Bananas	Yogurt	Salmon
Nuts	Beans	Tofu	Avocados
Yogurt	Whole grains bread	Salmon	Peanut butter
Tofu	Apples	Chicken	Seeds
Salmon		Beans	Olive oil
Chicken		Peanut butter	
Avocados		Seeds	
Beans			
Whole grains bread			
Apples			
Peanut butter			
Seeds			
Olive oil			

WORKSHEET 5

Identify which foods are complex carbohydrates and which foods are simple carbohydrates. Place a ✓ for all of the complex carbohydrates, and an X for all of the simple carbohydrates.

✓ Complex Carbohydrates   ✗ Simple Carbohydrates

Food		Food	
Rolled oats	✓	Soda	✗
Cookies	✗	Broccoli	✓
Apples	✓	White bread	✗
Fruit Juice	✗	White Pasta	✗
Lentils	✓	White Rice	✗
Quinoa	✓	Whole grain bread	✓
Doughnuts	✗	Whole Wheat Pasta	✓
Sugary Cereal	✗	Steel Cut Oats	✓
		Oranges	✓

WORKSHEET 6

"Sort the fat!" game: Place an X in the boxes for the fats your BRAIN would choose.

- Avocados ✗
- Olive oil ✗
- Walnuts ✗
- Salmon ✗
- Fried Chips ☐
- Packaged Pastries ☐
- Cheeseburgers ☐
- Pumpkin seeds ✗
- French fries ☐

WORKSHEET 7

Match micronutrient to food and then function:

- Vitamin C → Oranges → Immune system and healing wounds
- Magnesium → leafy greens, nuts, seeds → Muscles, bones, and energy
- Iron → Broccoli, spinach, kale, green beans → Healthy blood
- Vitamin D → sun/fish → Helps your blood clot
- Vitamin K → spinach, lentils, meat → Immune system, brain & bones

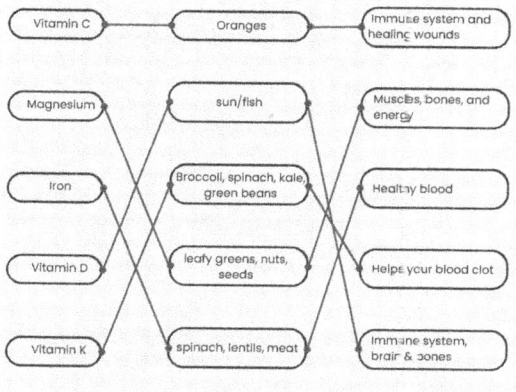

ANSWER KEY

WORKSHEET 9

Place a ✓ for which foods you microbiome would want you to eat.

- ☑ Blueberries
- ☑ Yogurt
- ☑ Rolled Oats
- ☑ Beans
- ☑ Onions
- ☐ Sugar free gatorade
- ☐ Doughnuts
- ☐ Gummy bears
- ☑ Garlic
- ☑ Asparagus
- ☐ Diet Soda
- ☑ Apples
- ☑ Lentils
- ☐ Potato Chips
- ☑ Quinoa
- ☐ White Bread

WORKSHEET 10

Match each food to the message it sends to your body:

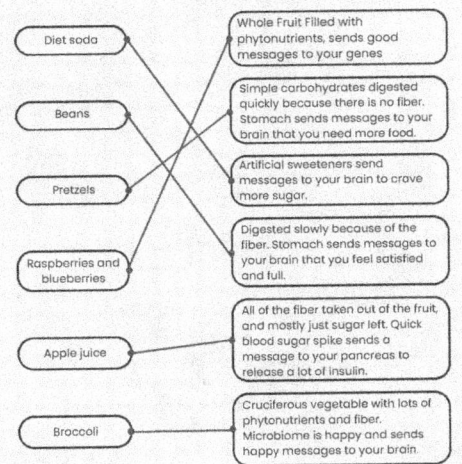

WORKSHEET 11

Compare the sugar, fiber, protein, sodium and ingredients for these 2 kinds of bread. Which has more of each? (Hint: Make sure to also look at the serving size, so you can accurately compare the two kinds of bread.)

White Bread:
- Sugar: 2.5 g/ Slice
- Fiber: 1.5 g/ Slice
- Protein: 2.5g/ Slice
- Sodium: 90 g/ slice
- Ingredients:

Whole Grain Ezekiel Bread:
- Sugar: 0g/ Slice
- Fiber: 3g/ Slice
- Protein: 5g/ Slice
- Sodium: 75g/ Slice
- Ingredients:

WORKSHEET 11

Were you surprised by the differences in these 2 types of bread?

Which one has more sugar per slice?
- White Bread

Which one has more protein per slice?
- Ezekiel Bread

Which one has more fiber per slice?
- Ezekiel Bread

Which one has less sodium per slice?
- Ezekiel Bread

How are the ingredients different between the 2 types of bread?
- The white bread has lots of ingredients that we would no find in a typical kitchen. The Ezekiel bread has fewer ingredients and are almost all whole foods

Circle which bread is a healthier choice. Explain why.
- Ezekiel Bread – More fiber, more protein, less sugar, less soduim, made with fewer ingredients

Why is it important to look at the serving size when comparing labels?
- It is important to look at the serving size so you can compare the same amount of food accurately.

WORKSHEET 12

Word find with names of sugar:

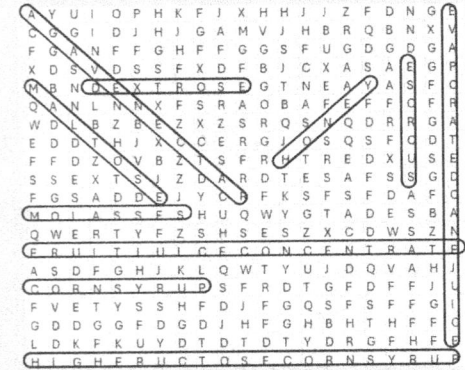

Agave Nectar   Honey   High fructose corn syrup
Corn syrup   Maltose   Evaporated cane juice   Sucrose
Dextrose   Molasses   Fruit juice concentrates

WORKSHEET 13

Word find with names for artificial sweeteners:

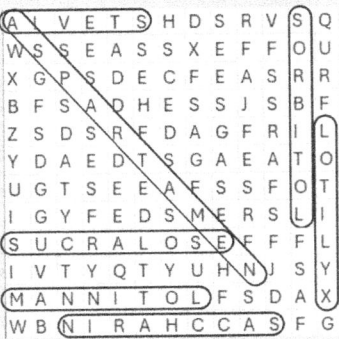

Words to find (Pronunciation in parenthesis):

Aspartame (AS-par-tame)   Xylitol (ZY-lih-tol)
Sorbitol (SOR-bih-tol)   Sucralose (SOO-kruh-lohs)
Mannitol (MAN-ih-tol)   Saccharin (SAK-uh-rin)
Stevia (STEE-vee-uh)

ANSWER KEY

WORKSHEET 15

Look closely at the ingredient lists for each of these foods.

- ✓ Place a check for the foods with ingredients you might find in a normal kitchen.
- ✗ Place an X for the foods with ingredients you don't recognize.

Vanilla Berry Yogurt Cup ✗   Oats ✓   Kid's Protein Brownie Bar ✗   Hummus ✓

Which 2 foods are the ultra-processed foods?
1. Vanilla Berry Yogurt Cup
2. Protein Bar

WORKSHEET 16

Compare the sample food labels:

<u>Frozen Breakfast sandwich</u> (with egg, sausage, and cheese)
<u>Homemade breakfast sandwich</u> (with Ezekiel English Muffin, egg, and avocado)

- Highlight total fat, saturated fat, trans fat.
- Look at the ingredients for added oils and fat.
- Identify which foods contain "brain-building fats" vs "not-so-great fats." Circle the healthy fats. Put an X next to the other "not-so-great fats."

Total fat: 26 g
Saturated fat: 10g
Trans fat: 0g

Total fat: 17 g
Saturated fat: 2.8g
Trans fat: 0g

Brain Building Fats:
Avocado and Pasture raised egg.

Not so great fats:
Palm oil, Soybean oil, Mono and Diglycerides, Fully Cooked Pork and Chicken Sausage Patty, Butter, and Lipolyzed Butter Oils, Cream

WORKSHEET 18

Using the labels below, sort each food into the correct category:

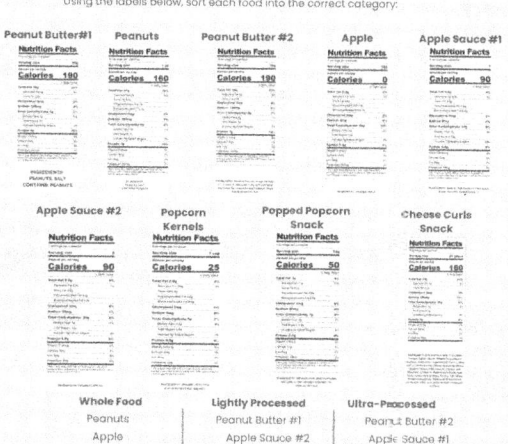

Whole Food	Lightly Processed	Ultra-Processed
Peanuts	Peanut Butter #1	Peanut Butter #2
Apple	Apple Sauce #2	Apple Sauce #1
Popcorn Kernels	Pop Corn Snack	Cheese Curls Snack

WORKSHEET 22

Compare the two foods and determine which is "Better for the Earth" vs. "Not as Earth-Friendly."

- Circle the food that is Better for the Earth.

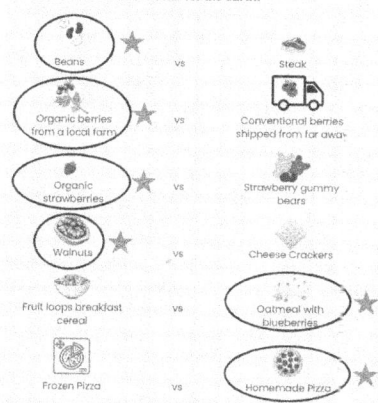

(Circled: Beans, Organic berries from a local farm, Organic strawberries, Walnuts, Oatmeal with blueberries, Homemade Pizza)

- Now put a star by the foods that are healthier for you

WORKSHEET 23

Circle which sources are a valid source to get nutrition information.

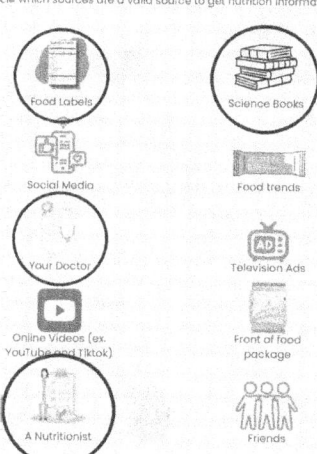

(Circled: Food Labels, Your Doctor, A Nutritionist)

Congratulations on Completing
"The Wonder of What We Eat Workbook!"

CERTIFICATE

OF
COMPLETION

Proudly presented to

_____

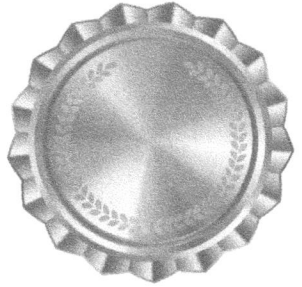

Dylan S.
DYLAN SHARMA

Ritu S.
RITU SALUJA-SHARMA MD

ABOUT THE AUTHORS

Dr. Ritu Saluja-Sharma, MD, is a double board-certified physician in Emergency Medicine and Lifestyle Medicine, a mom, and the founder of Head Heart Hands—a comprehensive, holistic wellness program for individuals and organizations.

After years of practicing Emergency Medicine on the frontlines of our healthcare system and seeing many of her patients suffering with diseases that could likely have been prevented, (and many which could potentially still be reversed), Dr Saluja-Sharma earned a second board certification in Lifestyle Medicine and created Head Heart Hands to help adults prevent and reverse disease by targeting ROOT CAUSES.

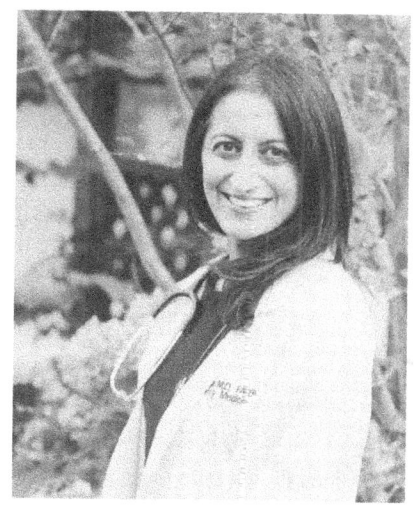

Her programs are designed to help participants lower their blood sugars, blood pressure, and cholesterol, increase their energy, improve their mood, decrease their pain, and improve their quality of life. As more and more adults have experienced incredible health transformations through her programs, they have frequently shared how they wished they had this help when they were younger. Teachers and principals have shared that they wished their students could learn the same tools and insights. Their experiences have inspired her to expand her focus to children, with the goal of helping the next generation build strong, healthy foundations—starting when it matters most.

Through her book, companion workbook, and cookbook, she's empowering a new generation to understand the power of food, build healthy mindsets, and fall in love with their bodies and the nourishment that fuels them. She is currently working to improve the health and nutrition curriculum in public schools and serves as an expert advisor on state-level curriculum standards.

Dylan Sharma is the co-author of The Wonder of What We Eat Workbook. He helped to design the kid-friendly activities and brought a student's perspective to the lessons. Dylan's interest in how food affects the health of the Earth and how the body works inspired him to help other kids learn in fun and relatable ways. When he's not reading (or writing) books, he enjoys running cross country, swimming and coding.

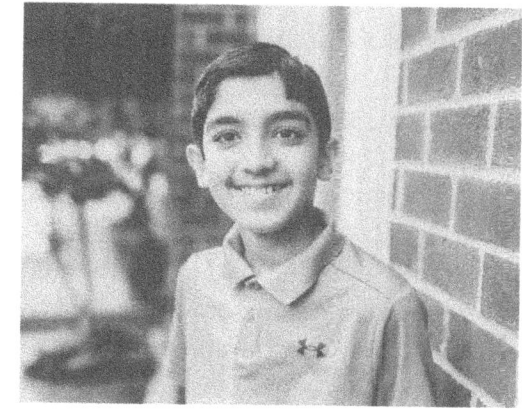

KEEP LEARNING, KEEP GROWING!

Loved this workbook? There's more to explore!

The Wonder of What We Eat Workbook is just the beginning. Keep the journey going with these two exciting companions:

The Wonder of What We Eat: How Our Incredible Food, Our Incredible Bodies, and Our Incredible Planet Are Connected
By Ritu Saluja-Sharma MD

The Wonder of What We Eat is a science-based, beautifully illustrated book that helps kids discover how food powers their body, brain, mood, and even the planet— all while building a healthy relationship with food, a positive body image, and a sense of empowerment over their own health.

Written by a physician and mom, this book is packed with:

- Eye-opening nutrition science (that even most adults haven't been taught) — like how food affects your microbiome, metabolism, genetics, and mood
- A fresh, empowering mindset around food and the body — replacing diet culture with a focus on nourishment, self-care, and seeing food as so much more than just calories or carbs
- Essential health literacy skills — including decision-making, goal-setting, and analyzing influences
- Encouragement and real-life tools — giving kids confidence and practical strategies they can use every day to expand their food choices, support healthy growth, and build habits that can help with picky eating and maintaining a healthy weight
- A supportive alternative to restrictive or shame-based messages — helping kids build a healthy relationship with food, understand their bodies, and make choices that help them thrive—now and for the future

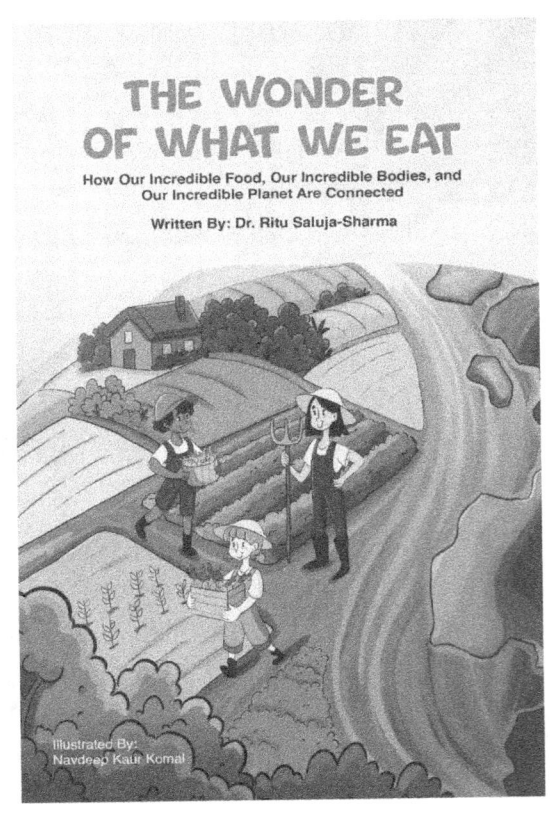

KEEP LEARNING, KEEP GROWING!

Loved this workbook? There's more to explore!

The Wonder of What We Eat Cookbook
By Ritu Saluja-Sharma, MD, Serena Sharma, and Dylan Sharma

The Wonder of What We Eat Cookbook is a beautifully designed, family-friendly recipe collection that brings the Head Heart Hands philosophy to life—helping kids (and parents) turn healthy intentions into delicious, shared experiences.

Written by a physician and mom, this cookbook offers:

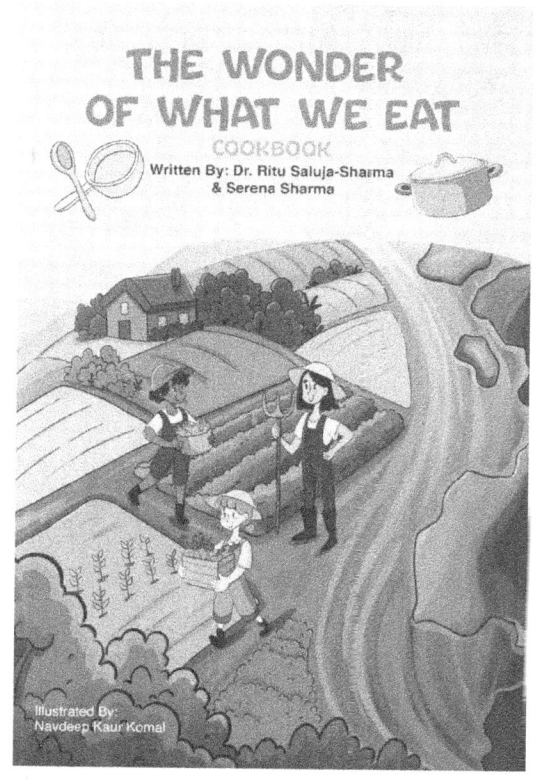

- Delicious, healthy, and nourishing recipes for breakfast, lunch, dinner, snack, and even dessert made with real ingredients—designed for families, to support growing bodies, sharp minds, and steady moods
- Kid-approved meals that even picky eaters can get excited about—so healthy food feels fun, not forced
- Step-by-step instructions that empower kids to cook on their own or alongside a parent
- Built-in learning moments, helping kids understand how food supports their health in ways they can see and feel
- A joyful, empowering experience for families, turning the kitchen into a space for connection, creativity, and confidence

Part of a 3-part system based on the Head Heart Hands method:
- The Book (Head): Empowers with knowledge. Builds a positive mindset about food and health
- The Workbook (Heart): Reinforces those lessons with reflection and real-life practice
- The Cookbook (Hands): Gives kids (and parents) the tools to apply it all in the kitchen

Want to help your kids build lifelong healthy habits, confidence in the kitchen, and a love for real, nourishing food? Make it happen—with *The Wonder of What We Eat Cookbook*.

FOR GROWN-UPS WHO WANT TO FEEL BETTER, TOO

If this book inspired you to think differently about food and health for your kids, you're not alone. Many adults reading this have asked the same question: "Where was this information when I was growing up?"

The truth is—it's never too late to start.
Dr. Ritu Saluja-Sharma, the author of The Wonder of What We Eat, is also the founder of **Head Heart Hands**.

What is Head Heart Hands?
It's an evidence-based, physician-created, proven, step-by-step program addressing all aspects of health including insulin resistance, inflammation, nutrition, and weight loss, but also stress, sleep, and mental health, designed to help you lose weight, increase your energy, and lower your blood sugars, cholesterol, and blood pressure in 12 Weeks.

Head: Step-By-Step Guidance and Mindset: Understand the Root Causes of our most common physical and mental health disorders. Learn how to target those root causes to help you lose weight, increase your energy, lower your blood sugars, decrease your cholesterol, and reduce your blood pressure, without medications.

Heart: Hope and Support: Our bodies are powerful and miraculous and are often capable of healing themselves. Improve your relationship with food, your body, and your health. Ditch dieting and instead focus on nourishment and self-care.

Hands: Tools and Reach: Implement positive changes into your life by using the many tools from this program, including meal plans, recipes, grocery lists, and challenges. Transcend the confines of hospitals and doctors' offices to meet you where you are- at school, at work, and at home.

Learn More
To explore online adult programs, corporate wellness, and hospital or school system partnerships visit headhearthandsmd.com. Or follow along on Instagram: @head_heart_handsmd

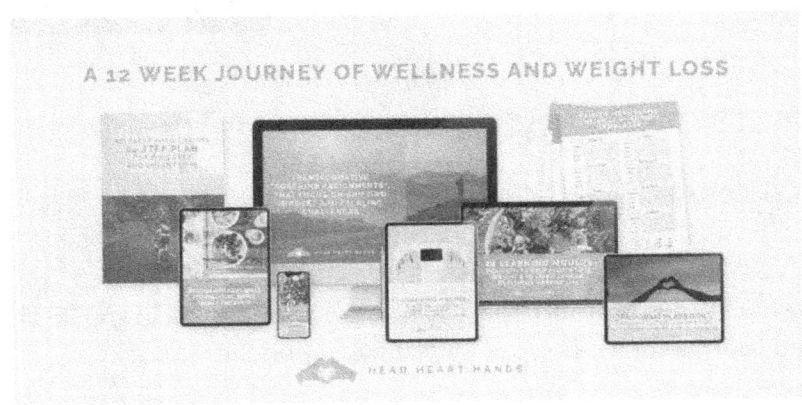

www.ingramcontent.com/pod-product-compliance
Lightning Source LLC
Chambersburg PA
CBHW080522030426
42337CB00023B/4595